D0507316

Things Are Going Great In My Absence

How To Let Go And Let The Divine

Do The Heavy Lifting

Lola Jones

Copyright © 2006-2012, Lola Jones

First edition, 2006

25th edition, 2012-2013

All rights reserved. Except for brief quotations in book reviews and articles, and as otherwise permitted by applicable law, no part of this book may be reproduced, used, stored, transmitted or displayed in any form, or by any means (electronic, mechanical, or otherwise) now known or hereafter devised—including photocopy, recording, or any information storage and retrieval system—without prior written permission from: Lola Jones. Contact admin@lolajones.com.

www.DivineOpenings.com

This book is not intended to replace your own inner guidance,
nor to provide or replace medical advice.

Published by Lola Jones.
Printed in the United States of America.

ISBN: 978-0-9859026-0-5

Acknowledgments and Appreciation

It would be impossible to name all the generous,
wise, and wonderful people who contributed to and shaped my life and spiritual
awakening, before and since Divine Openings. Those who've opened my heart and mind are many.
While most of the content of this book was channeled from within and was more profound and
effective than anything I'd ever learned from others, parts of it were catalyzed by great
teachers and powerful initiations. We create each other on this journey.
You created me to say what this book says.

A waterfall of appreciation and love to Russell Martin,
love of my life, who gave of his valuable time to advise, edit,
and proofread this final edition of the book,
and lend his enormous energy to it.

Appreciation to all the many of you who grace my life.

I love you.

IMPORTANT NOTE:

To insure the quality and purity of Divine Openings,

Lola Jones is the only person certifyng Divine Openings Givers at this time.

Things Are Going Great In My Absence:
How To Let Go And Let The Divine Do The Heavy Lifting

By Lola Jones

A dramatic awakening is happening on the planet right now. Human consciousness is expanding exponentially. Those of us out on the leading edge are experiencing a rapid flowering of enlightenment—right now, and we invite you to join us.

Receive an initiation to enlightenment, or a deepening of your enlightenment, as you read this book, gaze at the illustrations in it, and feel the Divine Presence in it—the Divine Presence that is in you. You will want everyone you know and care about to get this book, so they can share this bountiful experience with you and join you in this wondrous new world.

Whatever you want next in your life, this book will help you achieve it with more ease, Grace, and flow. You get help on two levels. You receive tools you can use to consciously make more powerful, effective choices. On another much more powerful level, you receive Divine Grace, which, by definition, is a gift you cannot earn. It lifts you higher than you could humanly lift yourself. Much of the process is effortless for you, as Grace does at least ninety percent of the work. Your ten percent is to learn how to let it in, and get out of the way. We show you how.

Once the Divine Presence in you is awake and walking this planet as *You*, once you are in the flow of life that supplies all wants and needs, creating the life you want is easy, fun, joyful, and exciting. Suffering, conflict, and struggle cease. Synchronicities become commonplace as you come together with people, resources, and events for mutual benefit and sharing of joy.

Once seeking is over and true living begins, you live in confidence, relish the moment, and create whatever you want. The "power of now" is a tangible reality rather than a wishful concept or book title. The past and the future have no hold on you, and loss, worry, and scarcity can no longer be found.

You are "unsinkable" when you live as your Large Self, and truly feel the power of who you are. Crime, government, heartbreak, money issues—nothing has power over you in this new paradigm. People around you literally transform because of who you are, and you never feel powerless to make a difference again, yet you know when to let go.

Begin right now to enjoy a more vital, personal relationship with your Creator, who is eager and waiting to co-create more closely with you to fulfill all of your heart's desires.

Lola Jones spent twenty-one days in silent retreat in early 2006, communing only with the Presence Within, and was initiated to give a special kind of Grace that activates awakening. She and other Divine Openings Givers give the initiation by touch, or they activate the Energy/Light/Intelligence by intention in group settings, or send it long distance. You'll experience it directly as you gaze at the art, read the words, and sit in the powerful vortex this book creates.

Lola's "job" is to get out of the way and let The Divine do the heavy lifting. She is "absent" from the process, even as she enjoys the blissful sensations of it. She also found that as The Divine in her woke up and she lived more fully as her Large Self, practical daily life continued to get easier and easier. Her Larger Self increasingly runs her life as her small self takes a back seat and relaxes, hence the title: *Things Are Going Great In My Absence.*

This is not only a chronicle of Lola's own awakening; it wakes up the Divine Intelligence in you. You learn how to receive it, what to expect in the process, how to get out of the way, allow it to be easier, and sustain it.

IMPORTANT
*On your first reading, this book **must***
*be read in order, **slowly**, from front to back.*
This is potent, powerful material, and you need to
absorb the instructions before receiving a Divine Opening,
and to understand the unfolding that follows. "Rushing"
reduces the results dramatically. It's not about
gaining knowledge. Experience it,
feel it, live it, bit by bit,
deeply.

As the energy accelerates, things change.
See www.DivineOpenings.com and join the email list
for updates, events, gifts, and inspiration.

If you ordered this book online you'll
receive a few automated email follow-ups.
Stay on that list to get free future
updates on the book.

You are about to enter a new reality.

Table Of Contents

Things Are Going Great In My Absence:
How To Let Go And Let The Divine Do The Heavy Lifting

How And Why I Wrote This Book

THIS BOOK FLOWED out of me very naturally and effortlessly after giving Divine Openings one-to-one and in groups for about six months. I didn't will it to happen; it willed me to write it. That's the way everything has gone these last few years. My body does what it wants to. It paints or writes when it wants to, or not. Sometimes I write all day and forget to eat. My old concept of ambition or motivation doesn't make much sense to me anymore. Things that used to seem important are not. Life lives through me. I mostly go along for the ride, watching the beautiful scenery go by, and enjoying the wonderful adventures on the way. It's the best ride of my life.

As the Divine Intelligence in you wakes up and takes over, as emotions arise, outer changes unfold, and the old reality unravels, this book helps your mind understand what's going on. You participated in the creation of this book. On some level you asked for it in your heart. The Divine Openings process doesn't require your mind's understanding, but your unfolding is accelerated when the mind cooperates rather than resists. This book retrains, guides, and soothes your mind during this time of change, when you're definitely out of your comfort zone. Until your inner knowing has flowered completely, it helps to have some help navigating the changes and integrating it all easily into your daily life. Until you are so clear you don't want any more outside guidance, stay open and let in the help until you truly don't need it. Please, always trust your own guidance and intuition over anyone's. This book embodies my experience helping thousands access their own truths and awaken to their own oneness with The Divine Intelligence within. It's unlike any book you've ever read, far beyond just intellectual concepts—it's an experience that alters your way of living.

The Light Emerges

WHILE GIVING DIVINE OPENINGS at a public event, going from one person to the next, touching each person for about two minutes, five of them reported seeing a brilliant white light through their closed eyelids as I stood in front of them. The normal expectation would be that someone standing in front of you would cause your field of vision to darken. (Try it!) But they were seeing my light body. When I am with people, one-to-one or in a group, a powerful vortex is created that activates or deepens their awakening and they realign more and more with the Pure Life Force that has always been inside of them. They awaken to what's not visible in the physical world.

None of this is to say I am special—it is to demonstrate that many of us human beings are quite literally becoming less dense and more purely light. The kinds of experiences you read about here are possible for you, and will eventually happen for those who stick with Divine Openings, learn to go within for your needs, and don't dilute it. I've initiated people around the world to give this enlightenment initiation, and they can do whatever they choose with it, but the standards to call it Divine Openings and be recommended personally by me on our official website are stringent.

Jesus and Mary were often depicted with a halo of light around their head or entire body. It was promised we would all one day be as they were, do the things they were able to do, and more. You will perform "miracles," which when you're in the flow of Life, become commonplace. What has been called "ascension" is the completed transformation of our bodies and minds so we become less dense. We are "en-lightening." Lightening up! Becoming more spacious.

As the light in each of us radiates more brightly, it becomes visible. We normally think of the function of eyes as receptors of light, because light goes into them. After their awakening begins, I notice clients' eyes lighting up—light is coming *from* their eyes, not just going *into* their eyes. In the first year after my initiation to give Divine Grace, I formally gave this enlightenment initiation to about seven hundred people, hands on, in small groups. That doesn't count the ones who have picked it up just by being in close proximity with me during daily life, or the many thousands who received it through the book and online courses. I've noticed it beginning to affect people after merely having dinner with them. If I see that happening, I offer this book so they'll understand the changes taking place, and so they can use their Free Will to reduce resistance to the Grace.

The Energy/Light/Intelligence of Divine Openings continually amps up; and as more and more people "light up," or "en-lighten," the whole collective consciousness of humanity lightens just a bit. People reading this book begin to see their own enlightenment reflecting in their families, friends, and co-workers. A rapid, spontaneous quickening, a chain reaction of enlightenment, takes place. I laugh as I tell people, "It won't be any big deal. It is who you naturally are. When you're there it will just seem normal." The unfolding of it is the real adventure. Enjoy every moment!

As you enlighten, you help humanity without doing or teaching anything. Those of us on this frontier brave the unknown and tame the wilderness for those who come after, and their way will be smoothed. Most won't know you helped them, just as you don't know the names of all the hardy American pioneers who paved the way to the New World for you. The ones who come along in your energetic footprints will benefit from your courage and foresight, and on the Larger level, they are You. This is your "joy," not your "work," and you came here eager to do it.

My friend related a story about a fellow karate master and teacher, a man's man who never studied metaphysics and was not on a spiritual path, who had a spontaneous enlightenment experience while he was alone in nature, in the mountains. Love enveloped him, tears flowed, and a sense of wonder and awe overtook him. He didn't know what was happening. Wondering who he knew that was weird enough to understand this, he confided in my friend, searching for explanations for this strange and unexpected change. They talked for two hours. He told of bringing his wife flowers for the first time in decades, upon which she inquired, "OK, who is she?" She thought he must have had an affair! He'd found love all right, but it was Divine, not carnal.

The karate master received Grace through a spontaneous opening. A precious few find it this way, or through seeking, or some spiritual path. Divine Openings gives you the opportunity to choose it now, rather than hoping it happens.

His state remains transformed, although I often help people who had such enlightenment experiences and could not sustain them until Divine Openings. One Buddhist (not a reader of this book) had a full-blown enlightenment experience that lasted for six months, until an encounter with his mother brought him crashing down!

This book gives not only the awakening, but the structure and support to maintain it. Our human mind and our outer world certainly don't validate or support it. I know of a few people who were committed temporarily to psychiatric hospitals when they had spontaneous, unplanned bursts of oneness and enlightenment. They marveled wide-eyed at the dancing leaves on the trees, and the light emanating from everything, and no one around them understood what was happening to them—and neither did they. That needn't happen when you undertake the process deliberately, with proper guidance and understanding. You can have a very functional enlightenment.

Once the awakening process begins, the most common early effect we hear is that anxiety disappears, replaced by a deep inexplicable knowing that all is well (the "peace that passes understanding"). The mind may at first want to control, define, or explain away Divine Openings, but as we grow accustomed to operating beyond the limited mind we relax into the Mystery.

Questions are answered most often from within, solutions arise effortlessly, with the occasional message or help coming serendipitously from someone or something outside. Striving stops, and there is a peace with the present moment and the "perfect imperfection" of our humanity.

There is still curiosity and desire (oh, yes, passionate desire) but no more frantic, lackful seeking. The urge to grow and expand is eternal, but the days of fruitless striving for it are over. Now you can stop working on yourself, healing issues, or needing someone to fix you.

I remind you several times to read *slowly* because people are so conditioned to read books in a mad rush, thinking the faster they can suck up the information, the sooner they can get on to the next book. That leads to shallow, futile, perpetual seeking. Sucking up information and speeding on is an unconscious tactic to avoid deep feeling and actual experience. Slow down to assimilate.

Even "advanced" people don't get everything the first time through this book. People tell me each subsequent reading is a next-level experience. That happens because your consciousness expands between readings unless you deliberately abandon Divine Openings or resist mightily.

Interestingly, you'll find that Divine Openings empties you out rather than filling your head with more intellectual knowledge. You get lighter, freer, and more spacious rather than more full of facts. You let more go, and toss more out. When you're tapped into the Flow of Life, you don't need to drag a lot of luggage on your journey, what you need shows up in the moment.

Divine Openings increases your capacity to tap into direct knowing. Spiritual and metaphysical theory, books, healings, and ancient texts are replaced with personal experience of The Divine, automatic evolution, direct downloads, and a living, breathing communion with a vast Intelligence.

Then what you choose to do with it and how you choose to live is completely up to you. The choices are limitless. I don't live by any spiritual stereotype, and you don't have to either.

Soon you will experience yourself "lighter."

What Happens With Divine Openings?

HOW DIVINE OPENINGS WORKS is beyond human intellectual comprehension. People have often told me they met me in a dream (sometimes I'm on my white horse!) right before they stumbled across my website. Our non-physical meeting prepared them to recognize me and Divine Openings in the physical. While I'm asleep my Large Self visits people and helps them, according to many emails I've received, but "I" am unaware of that, and I trust that's best. One of my greatest gifts is the ability to get completely out of the way and let the full power of Divine Openings use me without any need to understand, define, dissect, and so shrink it into something that would fit in a human brain. Nowhere in this book will you find a scientific rationale for it, because I don't care about such things. My playground is the Mystery out beyond science.

Since Divine Openings, my intellectual capacity has expanded dramatically, but it's not where my power resides. My gift is direct transmission of vibration, and direct knowing—words and intellectual concepts pale in comparison. That's why this isn't an ordinary book. A Mystery beyond words lights you up, opens you to larger realities, and changes your life (unless you resist really hard—I'm smiling real big right now.)

Then Divine Openings opens you up so you can let in the Grace that always is and always was raining down on you. It simply reveals to you what was already there and who you already are. It allows you to perceive what is real behind the illusion, to the degree you're willing to let it in (that ability increases with each reading of this book.) Most of what is real *is invisible and non-physical*, the opposite of the "physical reality worship" the world believes in. Love. Joy. Vibration. The Divine within you. The invisible begins to be perceptible. The physical world stops ruling you as you have direct experiences and tangible knowing of the non-physical world.

For years, the very word "God" made me cringe. We have a lot of baggage about this and other words due to all the fanatics, evangelists, and extremists who have used the word as an excuse to abuse and judge others. Now, I can finally say it again without tensing up. I'll use many other terms for God, but they are more cumbersome. Notice how the word God makes you feel. If there's a negative conditioned response, it will subside. No word can begin to describe the mystery and reverence I feel when I even think of the non-physical Source of All That Is, so for ease and brevity I use the word God a lot in this book. In my private life it needs no label—I am enfolded in it.

God cares about your ordinary life circumstances. As you develop a very close personal relationship with God, you'll impact your health, your finances, your love life, your family relationships, and your entire world in a very tangible, practical way. If you assimilate and practice what's in this book consistently——if you focus on Divine Openings for a year, and don't confuse yourself with other "stuff," you'll have anything you really want, in time.

I've taught many powerful systems before this, and Divine Openings has opened people up faster and easier than anything I've ever taught or done before. It has quite effortlessly removed obstacles and issues that neither the client nor I could perceive. You will find masses and layers of psychological conditioning lifting, and you may or may not ever know what it was. (You'll know if you needed to know.) You'll just find yourself feeling lighter, freer and happier. Your life blooms, and Divine Intelligence begins to express as your unique genius.

Before Divine Openings, in addition to teaching and helping others in personal and corporate settings, I had done way too many years of "clearing" and "healing" for myself. It was never-ending! It seemed the more I cleared, the more showed up to clear. Finally I said, "Enough! I want a path of joy, not work!" Divine Openings showed up, and massive change took place in my life without working on it at all. I felt more powerful and at peace than ever before. I also got healthier, more successful, confident and happy. No more processing, analyzing, or figuring it out.

Now it's so obvious looking back that "working on myself" had focused on what was wrong, and so created more issues than it relieved. When I let go and let The Divine do the heavy lifting, my life as a powerful creator began. I'm not saying Divine Openings is the only way; there is no one way for all. *I am saying it works.* Period. If I found a better way, I'd take it—but I have no reason to seek—the unfolding is now as natural as the cycles of nature, but much faster.

When you know, deep within, not just in your head, who you *really are*—a physical expression of a vast non-physical life force—you discover *all* of your old "issues" and limits were *illusory*; and slashing away at illusions is rather silly, isn't it?

There were many surprises. I had thought of myself more as a teacher, counselor, and enlightener, so I was at first quite surprised by the physical healings that occurred spontaneously during some of the Divine Openings, though people didn't tell me about their physical problem. I also give special physical healing sessions by telephone, as do other Divine Openings Givers. Some of them specialize in physical healing.

This book is the essential guide book for Divine Openings "Level One." As of 2011, there are three levels and six online retreats, plus the live retreats. Divine Openings keeps expanding, and I put most of the new material into sessions, online retreats and courses because I love the richness of multi-media and enjoy the total ease of updating the website constantly as the energies increase. In Five-Day Silent Retreats, I initiate others to give Divine Openings, and others take the 5 Day Retreat just for themselves.

Here are a few comments from people who have received Divine Openings. *DO NOT EXPECT THE SAME EXPERIENCE AS ANYONE ELSE!* Your unique experience is designed for you. I adore my own deep, subtle experiences. I also revel in hearing yours!

In their own words:

My seminars and treatments go easier and give both clients and myself more healing and pleasure, therefore filled up very well and expanded to Austria and South Africa even. My husband's work became more fun and better paid. We used to live (the five of us, I have three children) in a seventy-four square-meter flat and drive an eighteen-year-old car. Now we drive a five-year-old car with seven seats (so much space!) and live on 146 square meters with a stunning, big garden and neighbors better than we could have possibly dreamed them! We still walk through this beautiful, amazing house with our mouths open and stroll through the garden raving daily. And money, the major issue before, just keeps streaming in! Apart from these changes, I laugh a lot more, feel more peace, more serenity, more power, more love—I sometimes feel bursting of it all, it is so wonderful. I call it stretching the love and happiness muscles. Lots of love, — Gabriele, Germany

I have taken two of Lola's seminars, seven years ago, and recently. Both seminars made a HUGE difference in my life. I can honestly say that there were amazing shifts in my life after each course. —M.Z., recently on Oprah

I wanted more of God's spirit . . . so now here's more I can receive easier by Grace through Divine Openings, untainted by religious doctrine. Blessings, —Bev McCaw

I am seeing miraculous healings on a fairly regular basis! Blessed be! I am taking less insulin . . . I now know . . . I probably won't need it. It's all beyond good, obviously shaking me free of the past program. Thank-you! Lots of Love! —Steph

My business is profitable in "these" times! —LeAnn

That once a week Divine Opening is fifteen-twenty minutes of pure bliss that began to last longer and longer and longer. With much love and gratitude, —Teresa Anton, Pekin, Illinois

A warm tingly feeling spreads all through me, and in the morning when I wake, it's there again! Thank you so much for being there. —Elaine, Germany

I'm smiling too much, my husband doesn't know what to do with me! I have this amazing expectation that something big is about to happen . . . our financial/work headaches which were quite big now appear to be getting smaller and smaller. I am trusting Him in everything. What peace. Thank you, —Audrey, United Kingdom

Your work has the power of an atomic reactor. I was flooded with an incandescent internal light that was flooding thru me and the universe for quite a while. The next day I listened to one of the Diving In audios. I thought I was beaming off enough light to keep the east coast lit up for the remainder of the year. My dog was blissfully rolled over on her back and in sheer delight. She told me in doggie Yiddish, "who knew this Lola had such power, and from a recording no less." She sends ten energy licks of love for your face! I couldn't even sleep last night. —Love, Mark

Just wanted to share my appreciation of Divine Openings and say thanks. I have been reading the book, taking the course on-line and recently received a Divine Opening via conference call. Va va voom! Divine Openings has had such a powerful and yet subtle, gentle impact on my life. I used to dip down quite frequently and since coming to the website that first time, I find myself each day, staying steady or experiencing joy and more joy. —Laura

I am continuing reading your book and I am reading it slowly as well as trying my best to put into practice simultaneously whatsoever I read. I do feel that I am making a lot of progress, I feel my peacefulness is deepening and always happy all the time and very much energized and also I feel a mild blissful current running in my body most of the time. Love and Peace, —A. Punjabi, Philippines

Thank you for entering my life. —Conny, Malaysia. Age 51 years. wife, mother of 3 strapping boys, and corporate lady.

I'm now at the beginning of the online course, Week 1 and I already love it! Thank you for making this course reachable for many of us throughout the world! —Natasa, Macedonia

The book is so very helpful. I had an incident this morning where I went into judgment, and looked for the place in the book to learn how to be with and let emotions move through me. I made the request of the Divine and felt the compassion for myself and for others who get caught in it, and then I felt the release. It was just that simple. I do not even need to have a conversation with that person. Much Love, Many Blessings, —Cindy P, Austin, Texas

I can read your book only bits at a time because the energy is so strong. I have been developing my personal relationship with My Divine. I used to have that HUGE nebulous BIG SOURCE that was too big and abstract to contemplate as a personal friend. I do appreciate the 'structure' for my mind. —Beverly, United Kingdom

Hope you're doing well. I've been doing really great lately; you helped me out so much. I made several breakthroughs in the last two weeks. I finally let go of the stuff I was still carrying around from my ex-husband. I didn't know I still had that in me until I had a very vivid dream about him. This past Monday I had another dream that was just as vivid but was about my mother. I've been working on forgiving her all this week and I think I've done pretty well. I feel so much lighter and happier. My dreams have helped focus my attention to the people that I needed to forgive and I am very grateful for them. I've been able to stop the judging for the first time in my life. Again thank you so much, you are truly gifted. —Cindy F., Austin, Texas

Hi Lola, This is Sue from way down under in Australia. After my second Divine Opening, holy cow I felt a full range of emotions and the hairball I coughed up was HUGE. I went into a very dark place and I was angry, depressed, sad, lonely, and I was questioning everything and so much doubt crept in, the funny thing was while I was saying out loud "this is all crap, why am I bothering, etc, etc I found myself speaking to the Divine within ….Phew! I sobbed and swore and paced around my house and then I sat and dived right in to all of it! I asked the Divine to pull me up by the hand and guide me through the tough stuff, and for the next few days my emotions were all over the place ... and then all of a sudden the most beautiful sense of peace came over me and now I am feeling so happy and my cheeky, funny, silly child within has come out to play! Cool, I'm having fun! —Sue, Australia

The book has been everything I was looking for and more. So much has happened in the sixty days since opening it the first time that it would be virtually impossible to tell you everything. —Sallie B.

Awarenesses of how I've been resistant to receiving came up strongly. I asked God to soften that in me and then that "opening download" happened again immediately, and He told me, held me and showed me exactly what to do . . . I just experienced God in a much more intense way than ever before. I surrendered more than before and experienced a surging need to write even as I sobbed and yawned and released. I started in my journal and God wrote back. I've never experienced automatic writing before—what an awesome experience. Thank you for helping me remember my way Home as I'd gotten lost lately, and for helping me to access this amazing connection consciously in my daily life instead of just on retreats. Blessings to you, —Michelle Wolff

I felt a presence in the room, and could feel something 'opening', I can't exactly explain what opened up in me, but my more expensive work started selling. I sold one of my $2000 art pieces and the woman ordered two custom lamps too. —A. Broesche, Burnet, TX

My dog is so much better since the Divine Healing you sent. She had calcium deposits in her hips and was having difficulty getting around. Now, instead of limping and moaning and lying around on the floor and at the bottom of stairs she was avoiding, she is back to her old self—running, jumping on and off the furniture, going up and down stairs, and chasing her pal Shortie! We are overwhelmed with gratitude. Everyone who hasn't yet fallen in love with you, dear Lola, will, when they get your spirit, mind, body beauty treatment! —Erin, New Hope, Pennsylvania

I am focusing more powerfully at school. I can't describe the feeling I have when I connect with God now. I have no words for it. If I catch myself telling myself unproductive stories, I stop now. It is working. —Everett, high-school student, Pennsylvania

I was at your session two weeks ago. I just had what was probably the most incredible weekend of my adult life. I performed some of my music and was deeply heard. I received so much validation, encouragement——it was almost scary. My body is also changing, opening up, healing. I am so blessed by all of the synchronicity in my life right now. The Spirit is bringing all these things to me. I just have to try not to be afraid, to continue to breathe, and be willing to follow. Gratitude to you, sweet Lola, my cup runneth over. —Martha P., Georgetown, Texas.

I was hoping for some relief from the longstanding intense pain in my leg . . . I felt a tingling in my leg during the session, and the pain eased somewhat. Over the next few days, it became increasingly better, and is almost gone. I also felt some tingling in my injured shoulder. I had become resigned to that residual aching and restricted movement. That pain has gone, and I am able to move it much easier. I am so grateful for what I received. Sharon, The Woodlands,

Texas

I couldn't feel my body anymore and I lifted up out of it. I've always wanted to do this, and have meditated for years trying to. When it was over and I was back, I felt so good I didn't want to move, so I sat there for a long time. — Randy, Harlingen, Texas

This one is from a man who is initiated to give Divine Openings now. His day job is construction: Things are going very good with me and are constantly shifting into higher vibrations. Most places where I go or work are gradually raising in vibration, a few people at a time, even with the economy and oil prices. Some areas shift more rapidly than others depending on the resistance. —George Phon, California

After the first session, my endometriosis started healing, and now a week later, for the first time, I am not doubled over in pain with my brain not working during my period. I feel great, and this is amazing. It's a miracle for me and I can hardly believe it's happening. I have felt generally at ease all week, and for the first time in years my mind is not making up stories about what could go wrong. —Michele, Austin, Texas

I have been seeing myself from outside my own body, and at first not recognizing it as me. I am in bliss much of the time, quietly smiling. Things just don't bother me. I am starting to exercise and take better care of myself. —Cindy, Houston, Texas

Three years ago, I lost everything, husband, house, career... and although life went on and friends took care of me, I would wake up in anxiety every morning. The morning after my first Divine Opening, I woke feeling calm and light. I kept waiting to see if the anxiety would strike, but it hasn't come back. —Lynn Andrews, Austin, Texas

THAT is good stuff! I felt tension in my shoulder, jaw, and heart area release, and my head felt as if it was literally expanding. Things are getting wild. Much joy. XOXO. —Laura Graf, Singer, Austin, Texas

Others have had spontaneous openings in their ability to let in love and find relationship happiness, deeper communion or oneness with God, quieter mind, and less stress. Most people quickly lose their fears, worries, old blocks, and limitations. Relationships are set right. Creativity explodes. New lives are begun. Defenses and old hurts are dropped and, overnight, new love is found. Some begin to exercise without will power, achieve clarity of mind, and build their businesses with more ease and enjoyment. We've received thousands of emails, but don't compare your experiences to others' experiences, because yours will be unique and perfect for you. The subtlest experiences, like most of mine are, can be the most powerful.

People vary in their speed of awakening. Some of you will awaken quickly and see the results in your life and in those around you immediately as you read this book. Others "get it" on their third or fourth reading of the book. Many find an online retreat, a live Divine Opening, or a session series puts it in a higher gear. Everyone goes to an even higher level from a live Divine Opening because the vortex is more powerful live, and we can help you see your blind spots. Everyone goes higher through the online retreats because of the audios and videos: your habitual vibration is retrained as you spend time in this vortex of higher resonance.

The Divine does the heavy lifting. Just let go and get out of the way.

Divine Openings Givers Are "Specialists"

WHEN I WANT computer help, I go to a computer expert. I may ask within and get guidance on who to call or where to look, but I let humans help me. Sometimes the computer has fixed itself, but many times it comes through an intermediary—a person, book, website, or thing. In creation, there are experts we call upon for their specialties.

I am a specialist in evolution. New, raw, evolutionary waves of Energy/Light/Intelligence "vibrate me." They are not verbal and could never be fully explained verbally. I am a natural transformer and translator who makes the Energy/Light/Intelligence accessible for other humans, especially in practical life applications. Most of it is done vibrationally, although the words do help the conscious mind along. That's as much as I need to know about it. I care nothing for esoteric discourse or theory. If it doesn't help people practically, it's utterly uninteresting to me.

Each of has our own genius. You are a genius at something, and Divine Openings helps you discover and unfold it. So while I think it's ideal for you to become primarily inner-guided, I'm a specialist who can catalyze your awakening, speed and smooth the process, and support it ongoingly if you need that. I'm a specialist in bringing Heaven to Earth, bringing it down to practical, everyday life rather than just showing you how to float around in the spiritual realms. I won't tell you one thing about what you should do, or how you should live after your awakening—I just point to the door marked "Freedom," you walk through, and then it's your world!

Once awakened, most people come visit the website like you'd visit an old friend, even if they don't *need* to, to read the quote of the day, a new article, get inspired and uplifted, take a course, bask in the powerful field of resonance, or be in community. Wanting inspiration and compatible energy is natural—I need it too. So much of the input we get from the world isn't uplifting and doesn't support this awakened life we've chosen to live. I don't "do" mass media at all except selected music and movies. Instead, we created our own compatible and supportive "world" at www.DivineOpenings.com.

How To Get The Maximum From This Experience

LET GO OF the need to mentally figure it out. Your mind cannot fathom Divine Openings, and wants to stuff it in some existing category. That holds you back. Every time you hear your mind say, "I already knew that," STOP! Are you living it fully? How could you get it at a new level?

Commit to play with, feel, and experience it. Go for it with all your heart—but gently, reading slowly—integrating it step by step into your daily life.

You have Free Will. Even Grace cannot take that away, nor would we want it to. You each come to Divine Openings with varying degrees of willingness and openness. Some people release resistance quickly—some let go more slowly. Some cling to things they know are holding them back. Some have strong resistance to feeling, and that slows them down, but it does not stop them.

Some find their attitudes shifting noticeably in a week, many more see a big difference in a month, all of you will within a year—if you commit, enjoy, and don't dilute it with other stuff.

Sometimes people with several decades of spiritual experience move more slowly than the beginners. The beginners' minds aren't so overcrowded. If the "experienced" people think they know it already, they invariably miss it by thinking, "I've already heard that." But this is beyond any *words or concepts*. And you're ready for a higher, next-level truth now.

Some people searched for so long that searching became an addiction, an end in itself, and the original reason for it was forgotten. You may have become discouraged. You may have felt the search was endless. Now you can experience God instead of seeking God. If you want it all, let go of everything. Ditch the second-hand concepts, cliché New Age truisms, and all that stuff someone or some book told you. Open up space for direct knowing from within. Come to Divine Openings with an empty mind, the curious, eager, and open mind of a child.

Truth is radically different at different levels of consciousness.

Write here, or on the first pages of your notebook: Today's date _____
What you want—the whole list, including what you think is impossible.
What you want that you've "worked at" but hasn't happened.
What your challenges are.
What you want to let go of.

What you want to let in and how you want to feel.

Sign and date here to commemorate this happy day: _____
Come back to this page (or your notebook) at three, six, and twelve months and notice the changes in your life. Write them here:

Did the things you wanted change as you lived into your authentic Self? One thing is certain—no matter how it plays out, or in what form, you can have what your *heart* has truly desired for so long.

Dancing Lessons From God

WHEN I TOLD a friend this book was about what happens when the small self gets in the back seat and the Large Self drives, he teased, "So then the story will have some exciting car chases and rollovers?" I laughed, "Life is a *drama-free zone* once the Large Self is driving." My life wasn't always drama free, but once you dive into your own true Being and start living as your Large Self, instead of drama you'll have adventures, but ones you enjoy, and ones you create on purpose.

The best things in my life had always come naturally. Our Large, Unlimited Self knows what we want more than we ourselves know, and the best form in which to deliver it. But I still didn't completely let go and let my Large Self do the driving until I was past fifty, when Divine Openings arrived. I need no goals now, yet things move faster, and there's more magic than ever.

A number of years ago, I had a big mid-life hormone crash, and a lucrative corporate training and consulting career, and all my motivation, vaporized almost overnight. I stopped my spiritual teaching as well (I was sick of mere words, and their limitations), and became an artist for two years to rest in the creative silence and restore my soul. I thought, "I'm middle-aged and burned out. I can't rebuild again." But in the barren cold of winter, unseen underground forces are always at work, gathering, building. For some time I had sensed something big was coming—as usual, something I clearly could not plan for or predict. What came was beyond my wildest imaginings.

In December 2005, I had never even heard of regular humans being able to initiate enlightenment with a mere touch or intention, and by March 2006 I was on a plane to India to become initiated to do just that. Many lifetimes of being an enlightener were reactivated instantly, enabling me to activate the enlightenment process in other people. Emotional, mental, spiritual and physical suffering are relieved without working on them. Life issues, even those they had worked on for decades, resolve easily.

I never dared believe I could do such things, although the desire to do this was born when I first laid eyes on an enlightened master in 1985. "But get real," I told myself, "you can never be what he is." The years went by and I forgot my "foolish" desire. If you had told me then that nineteen years later I would possess this power, it would have been beyond my wildest dreams. And many of my clients and students have much wilder experiences than I do! I joke about my science fiction life, but the funny thing is, now it seems quite normal.

A little of the teaching I was given in India was a good fit for me; the rest did not resonate with me at all, especially the giving of all the power to the gurus, so I left those parts behind. It was quickly clear that I needed to, with appreciation, break with the organization in India and continue the evolution through direct Divine guidance and direct knowing, for which I have a gift. The power actually increased without the buffer of the teachers, which took a bit of getting used to at first. Then it became my passion to help people "go direct" to their inner teacher.

Some of what I teach came to me intuitively as long as twenty years ago, and much of it is up-to-the-minute inspiration from within. Some is influenced by beloved past teachers. Most comes from The Presence expressing through me, as pure vibration, touch, words, art, and music.

Different people are drawn to different teachers, because different teachers are called to say it in different ways. Divine Openings of course isn't the only way, but it works better than anything I've ever known, it ended my seeking, and has awakened many.

I've found most people need something to wrap their mind around early in this awakening process. A really effective method of conscious mind retraining was absent in the organization in India, and many still struggled afterward in their daily lives. I developed ways to accelerate, support, and ease the awakening, make it work in practical life, and sustain it.

I somehow knew from day one in India that I'd develop the ability to initiate "enlighteners" despite the teachers in India saying only they could do that. There's a deep knowing that I've done that in many previous lives, and I had absolutely no doubt. Within nine months of coming home, I stabilized, established Divine Openings locally, and wrote this book. Then I knew it was time to initiate other Divine Openings Givers. I announced the first Five-Day Silent Retreat, and people registered without question. Many people know very quickly if it's for them as they read this book.

The initiation to *give* Divine Openings is much more intense than the level of initiation you receive from this book. That first year I initiated people to give Divine Openings the intense Energy/Light/Intelligence flowing through me dominated my entire being, challenging my nervous system's capacity to handle it. I couldn't do anything else for about two weeks before, during, and after the Five-Day Silent Retreats. Physical stamina dropped, I couldn't do my other work, nor add two and two (my left brain barely worked.) All my mind, body, and spirit's resources were used by the initiation process, much as running a very large program on your computer bogs down other programs running at the same time. It wasn't hard, it just required *all* of me.

It was similar to being wired for 110 volts of electricity, and trying to run 220 volts. Now, the continual new incoming Energy/Light/Intelligence is more easily assimilated, as my "wiring" has been upgraded tremendously. I can now function more normally when I'm initiating others, although my human self is often somewhat "absent." Things do go great in my absence.

You'll get to the real "meat" of this book halfway through. It gets deeper and better as it goes. I recommend you read slowly and don't skip ahead for good reason. Let the vibration prepare you step by step as you read and feel. Notice any impatience. If you're saying, "I'm advanced, so I can skip ahead," STOP! That will cause you to miss important things. Past experience is best left behind. "The last shall be first, and the first shall be last," and "You must come as a little child" now make total sense to me. It means you must let go of all you know to get "into Heaven." That's what I did in my twenty-one days—I let it *all* go.

The End of Effort

AS I GIVE Divine Openings, and initiate others to give it, I completely let go to my Large Self. The pure Divine in me uses my body, mind, voice, and hands while I relax into the blissful sensation of it. Delicious, causeless tears of love might stream. We are the body of The Divine when we get out of the way. It's not work. My trying to *do* or *know* too much would seriously diminish the power and results of it.

It has been said that the coming Golden Age is the end of effort—a return to the easy, effortless flow of Life, a return to The Garden, where we're aligned with The Divine such that we are led in every moment, surely, swiftly, accurately to what we want and need. The "efforts" I make, and even my challenges, feel more like play, creativity, and productivity than what I used to think of as "work."

Frankly, India was never on my travel wish list. I've never studied eastern religion, and was thoroughly uninterested in India before I was called from within to go. I have no desire to go back. I know I've lived many, many past lives there, but I'm firmly centered in the present, I have zero interest in history or past lives. What I do and give was in my heritage—a gift that since its full activation now requires no effort, no study, and no work. I felt I had finally come home after wandering in the desert—home to my own heart, my own Source.

The light of the Divine has always been there; enlightenment brings the ability to see it. All your power is right here, in the present moment. All you need to know is available here and now. Seeking too much intellectual knowledge is a mind trap—you can never get enough. I've never seen it liberate anyone—ever—although I've watched so many try! Understanding and knowledge are the booby prize, the small self's way to keep us chasing after more, more, more information.

Mankind has wandered far from home. The passing age has been one of diverging from The Divine, of man exploring his own Free Will, guided by his logical mind instead of The Divine Intelligence within, buying into the illusion that the physical world is immutable and all-powerful— often at the cost of losing his own happiness and fulfillment. It's been a grand drama. We're proud of our struggles and suffering. We make heroes of those who were lost and then found, as any movie plot demonstrates. Struggle is highly valued and rewarded.

We have taken off in our airplanes and pointed straight into a strong headwind, straining our engines, pushing with all our might against the flow that would carry us with a fraction of the effort if we allowed it. If anyone were to say, "Ummm, you could just turn downwind and go with the natural flow," we would say, "But where's the glory in that? I'm strong. I want to succeed my way and prove it." And it is true that everyone from our parents to our clients and employers cheer us on when we work hard, when we struggle and fight, sweat and strain. "Good work! You're such a hard worker! You have such perseverance! You overcame adversity."

Here's the good news. Finally, we're remembering that the adversity we were so busy overcoming… was our own creation. Now we can just as easily create our lives with less struggle, and so have very little to overcome. We can use that energy for more fun, proactive, and rewarding adventures and creations.

The world can't be changed from the outside, but what's in each human can be awakened. No amount of teaching, policing, regulating, forcing, controlling, or punishing has succeeded in changing the world. Such a shift can only come from within. When people are governed by the heart and guided by their Inner Source, no external regulation whatsoever is required.

Einstein said that no problem is solved from the same consciousness that created it. I show people how to stop trying to solve problems on the physical plane and to instead shift their energy and focus their intention, aligning them with Pure Divine Presence. From this new perspective, soon the old problem simply isn't there! An experience of mine illustrates this. I have to reach way back to find such a dramatic example of struggle. It's simply not a part of my reality anymore.

Many years ago, when my vibration was a lot lower, a Houston lawyer decided not to pay me twenty-four thousand dollars he owed me. He knew I would probably sue him after many months of sending past due notices and calling his office to no avail. So he sued me first, which put him in control of a game at which he excelled. I was fearful, as I had invested months in the project and needed the money, and was afraid he'd sink me financially with the legal expenses he could force me to run up. I hired an attorney, went over and over the facts obsessively, made the Houston lawyer the bad guy, and laid awake nights quaking, obsessing over what to do, how to fight him, and how terrified of him I was.

After about six months (I was a little slow back then) I finally turned it over to The Divine and asked for dream guidance. Soon I had a dream in which a formal, authoritative man in a tuxedo gave me the keys to a very large white automobile. It was so huge that I could barely see over the steering wheel. As I drove out of the car lot, I stopped to ask the man questions. He simply waved me on, ordering, *"Just drive away."* I woke with a whole new perspective; in that dream my consciousness had been instantaneously adjusted to a place of peace and wellbeing. From that day on, I never thought about the situation again except to recount the fantastic dream of the white car. In my thoughts and speech I never made the Houston lawyer the bad guy again. In my heart, I was resolved with him, compassionate to him and his own demons. I knew it was over, long before there was a shred of physical evidence. Feeling a little better and vibrating a little higher always precede improvement in the physical world. I just "drove away" as directed, focused on other things, and moved ahead with life.

I heard nothing for another six months. One day my attorney called with a settlement offer of five thousand dollars. I confidently said "no" and once again forgot about it. Months later, another call came, this time with a settlement offer for twelve-thousand dollars. This time I said yes, since the money would be timely, and it would all finally be over and resolved—that was worth thousands to me. In that past state of consciousness, that settlement was the best victory I could manage, and it was pretty good. In today's consciousness I would have said no to that settlement, confident that I would get it all in time, or more. I have none of that old victim vibration left in me, and don't find myself playing victim roles at all anymore. Victimhood is seductive because the victim gets to be right—the innocent *good guy.* You'll learn it's not worth it.

At each chapter throughout that saga, my way of dealing with it shifted with each elevation in consciousness, and as Einstein predicted, the solution existed in a completely different consciousness than the one in which the problem was created. My life is drama-free now, and I'm clear that I am the author of it all. Today and going forward, I'd be unlikely to manifest a lawsuit. That can only happen from a lower vibration, or if I ignored or resisted my own guidance.

Today, when I urge students just to "just drive away" they get the metaphor. Do you need to clear, heal, process, analyze or fix your past? No. Just drive away, eyes forward. Don't worry about how—Divine Openings helps you do it. Just read on.

Just drive away.

A certain way of Being produces certain kinds of doing, which produces vibrationally matching results. Most of the world throws action, time, money, and work at a problem instead of shifting the way of *being* that produced that problem in the first place. Action wasn't helping the legal problem— it was actually making it worse. Shifting my own *being* worked. When your business is not going well, an action approach would be to work harder and longer, get new employees, talk to creditors, or change your processes. But it would be more effective to *first* change the inner state that caused those past results. "Be" clearer, then you'll "do" more effective things, then you'll "have" better business results. Align energy and intention first -- materialization follows.

"Be" it first, then you'll "do" different things, and then you'll "have" different results.

Most of the world thinks that if they had more money, things would go better, and then they could be happy. But that's backwards. That's "have, do, be." The reverse is true: if you could "be" happier and more centered, you would "do" better, and then you'd "have" more money. This book is not going to ask you to "do" anything different. You'll allow your true inner being to emerge until you are *being* your Large Self, then you'll watch your actions and thoughts flow naturally from that. Then your life and circumstances will shift around to fit who you newly are. They must, and they will, without effort.

Since I mentioned materializing money (a highly charged and misunderstood subject), consider this. When you can consistently "be" happy, your joy won't be dependent on how many dollars you have in the bank anyway. When you're in the abundant flow of life, what you need comes to you when you need it, sometimes without needing money. When you feel secure in that knowing, the number of dollars you have stored up doesn't matter, although indeed you may find your savings growing. When you don't feel secure, no amount of money makes you secure. You've seen millionaires who cannot rest or play, and are in constant fear of losing their millions. And they can lose it. You can feel completely secure with an empty checking account living in a cozy trailer home when your relationship with your powerful Divine Self is strong.

Money is much less important than claiming your Divine creative ability. Some of you will use this book and your creative ability to make lots of money. Some of you won't care so much about money once you're happy, or you won't need much. It's your reality—your grand, creative experiment—and you get to choose. Once you're awake, you'll know what's really true for *you.*

The phenomenon that we call our reality is not the solid, concrete thing we think it is. The translating mechanisms of our senses and our brain make it appear solid. My changes in my perception of the lawyer and the lawsuit produced changes in my physical reality. If you'll focus first on your consciousness, vibration, and state of being, materials issues will clear up.

Ten years ago I worked with people to change their thinking and their perception of things, and then their relationships would improve, their incomes would rise, and they were happier and more successful. This was all good, and it was state-of-the-art at the time, but there are now more profound ways to change reality than working on details like thoughts and perceptions.

Divine Openings doesn't work on details at all. It doesn't need to because it works at the meta-level (very big picture), and causes quantum evolutionary leaps at every level of your being simultaneously.

It literally upgrades you, reconnecting DNA strands, hooking up new evolutionary strands, restoring lost connections to the earth and other dimensions, and activating your light body. Most people feel a tingling or expansive feeling after some number of Divine Openings, from the book, but even more so with live contact with the field of resonance. Sit quietly after each Divine Opening to fully feel the nuances. You could *feel nothing* and still have dramatic changes in your life within weeks or months. Stop taking score. Notice what's better in your life. Journal only about your successes and what you appreciate, and stop talking about and journaling about problems. You get more of what you focus on because your focus has enormous creative power in it.

Divine Openings changes you on all levels, without work.

If this sounds fantastic, there is more to come, much more. The evolution that will occur in mankind in the coming decade is beyond our wildest imaginings, because evolution has been speeding up exponentially and will continue to do so. Imagine if you were a cave man walking our streets, observing our computers, planes, and cars. It would be mind-boggling. Even in the 1800s, could you have wrapped your mind around television, space travel, the Internet, cell phones, video conferencing, and jet airplanes? Our current reality is soon going to seem as primitive in retrospect as the cave man's seems to us now. From the limitations of today's consciousness we have no way of conceiving of what's coming because it will take tomorrow's vastly evolved consciousness to create that emerging future.

More has happened in the last fifty years than formerly happened in many hundreds of generations. These days you don't have to die to get a fresh new life. You can just start a new one right here—if you're willing to let go of even the best of what you knew before. I often joke about the many lives I've already lived in this body, and more are coming.

Divine Openings has expanded rapidly since my twenty-one days of silence, and thankfully, it continues to, sometimes weekly! I often re-read this book because the Large Self *me* that writes and teaches is ahead of the everyday me, so it's continually amazing that I "expand" from reading my own book! Your Large Self will always be out ahead of your smaller, more limited self, calling you forward into your heart's desires. Go and it feels good. Resist and it hurts. It's that simple.

My intention is that you establish your own main line to your inner guru. Sure, many people in your life have gifts for you. They say or offer something at just the right time. They open doors for you, or add richness to your experience. The Divine Life Force lives and expresses through all of us. Be open-minded, but be very picky about what you let in—there's so much stuff out there that doesn't work, isn't helpful, and that can pull you off track. Keep yourself surrounded by uplifting people, things, events, and websites like www.DivineOpenings.com. But if anything tempts you to go back to seeking, or to give your power away to anything outside you, think carefully, it is a crucial choice. This book keeps guiding you back inside yourself, over and over.

It used to be a lot of work to control our negative, runaway minds and our wild emotions in order to change our lives. Soon you'll have an easier job of it. A woman told me recently, "The little devil inside my head is just gone!" That was a gift of Grace. The Divine did the heavy lifting.

You will learn to use your Free Will wisely, but it isn't work, it's just paying attention. There's no "working on yourself" or "processing" in Divine Openings. You just *stay awake.*

I know many of you have a strong desire to make a difference on the planet, but take plenty of time get yourself completely free first. You can exhaust yourself doing it the old way. You're going to discover ways to change the world that you cannot now imagine—it's different than you think, and you're going to like it. Fasten your seatbelts, place your tray tables in their upright and locked positions, and enjoy the ride.

It's An Experience, Not A Concept

TALKING, READING, AND HEARING about spiritual things are often barriers to actual inner knowing. But you're about to have a direct experience of The Divine within you. This invisible Larger aspect of You will soon become a normal everyday part of your life.

A Divine Opening can be activated in any number of ways. When we see people one to one we give Divine Openings by touch for a minute or so, or I sometimes give "Divine Mother hugs." When it's a large group we cause the Divine Openings by intention from the front of the room, without touch. It's just as powerful. The Divine Openings can also be activated through art (as in this book), music, by phone, or by any means imaginable. Divine Openings work by long distance too. Sometimes the group closes their eyes while Lola sings a song that carries the Divine Opening. In the Five-Day Silent Retreat, we use a very powerful form, given by gazing into your eyes: The Divine looking at The Divine.

You can only get it by experience—it's not something to learn, figure out, or understand with the mind—so it's best to leave the mind out of it. Some people do best with support and coaching, since it's beyond the mind's comfort zone, and your mind may resist it because it disrupts your ordinary reality. The mind can't stop it entirely, but it can slow you down.

Divine Openings indeed activates your enlightenment, and helps you let in more Grace. It's all a matter of time, and the timing is for The Divine and you to decide. If you want results more quickly, relax, read the book slowly, deliciously, and repeatedly, but don't make it into work.

Intellectual, analytical people do better if they can let go of thinking, and feel everything instead. (Our many online offerings provide extra help.) Simple villagers have become fully enlightened with one blessing by a master, because there was less mental clutter, and fewer ego constructs and spiritual pretenses to shed to restore that most simple, natural, and innocent state.

People often tell me all the spiritual books they've read, the gurus they've lived with, and all the things they know. I'll teasingly say, "Then you don't need me." They admit they're still not happy or fulfilled, or it's not "working" on the practical level. Perhaps they're still struggling with money, or emotions, or relationships. Let go of past knowing to go higher. Slow down. Stop working at it.

Enlightenment is not an intellectual process, and intellectual processes are counterproductive to it. You cannot mentally figure it out. Understanding is the booby prize. The mind cannot take you there no matter how many books you read and how much religious or spiritual knowledge you accumulate. Enlightenment can't be earned by hard work or service. You can't rush or control it. Nor can you get it by being good, doing good works, or "being spiritual." Divine Grace can give it in a heartbeat.

Divine Openings doesn't even fit in any "spiritual" box. Leave all your old concepts of God, religion, and spirituality behind and have a pure, powerful, and authentic experience. You wouldn't eat secondhand food. Don't ingest second-hand experiences of God, no matter who said it. You'll move faster if you open up to pure, new experience, and let go of everything you knew before. People ask what was most powerful about my twenty-one days of silence: "I got empty."

Mental and intellectual understanding is the booby prize.

Divine Openings so profoundly changes you, and so radically shifts reality, that one week after a session many had to strain to remember the huge problem they came to me with. It was that "gone." That often happens—people often just go on to their new reality and forget they were ever in the old one. They get so busy living they don't have much interest in the past, how they got into the problem, and what got them out. You'll know you're free when there's little interest in the past and no interest in retelling past dramas and problems anymore. This is the new paradigm of living in the now. The hazy past seems unreal. Do share with those you love before you forget how you got free! They don't know how to get where you are, and telling them *intellectually* to "do this or that" won't work, and can really frustrate them. Talk just never does it. Share the book and website with them and give them the same advantages you had.

The Small Self Lets Go

SOME CALL IT the ego, but I call it the small self so you can see it fresh and not make it "bad." Small self is simply that more narrowly focused, less knowing aspect of us that thinks it is separate from God, other people, and the Creation. It's the part that might resist the Grace that would carry us with ease. It is fearful, scarcity-oriented, defensive, habit-driven, and has created all kinds of compensatory strategies to protect against things that it itself has created. It believes that life is basically a struggle against something "out there." The small self is much like an astronaut would be if no Command Central back in Houston gave the Larger view, and if there was no computer on board the craft that could calculate more than the limited brain and senses could offer. He'd be lost and adrift out in space. That smaller self thinks it's just a brain in a body. It doesn't have to be our limiting factor anymore, and you don't have to get rid of it or worry about it; the small self relaxes, opens up and evolves. To speed your awakening, embrace it rather than resisting it.

When we rely only on our senses and those things we can see, feel, touch, smell and taste, we are without the greater guidance of the Large Self. Divine Openings reunites us with our Larger Self, which has that broader perspective and knows the bigger picture of our lives, the world, the Universe, and the other dimensions. Small self is the lesser part of us that allows us to narrow down and have the experience of being human individuals, but we're always encompassed by and enfolded in the greater Large Self. Any boundary between the Large and small self is imaginary.

Your small self goes through a short or long process of letting go. As you embrace and soothe it, it gets in the back seat and enjoys the ride while the Large Self flies the plane. Life goes more smoothly and there is more joy when the Large Self is in the driver's seat. The small self can know fleeting pleasures, but it can't know joy until it has relaxed into the care of the Large Self.

This book guides you as you awaken, so you may now relax. When the small self stops struggling and gets on the wave the Large Self has created, we enjoy surfing Life. The ride is for fun, not to get somewhere or prove our worth (you'll discover your worth is a given) .

Support For Your Journey

THOSE OF US living the Divine Openings life belong to a collective consciousness that exists beyond Earth's consensus reality, and we celebrate, support, and uplift each other in our explosion into bright new possibilities. We commune on many levels, even if we live across the world. As I've already shared with you I am constantly in awe and wonder at how we are One, such that we meet in dreams and other dimensions, assist each other, and "know things" across distances. Past Five-Day Silent Retreat participants can feel the energy of current retreats building. They often contribute on other planes or dream they're here helping.

Our Divine Openings collective is tremendously powerful, and it continues to rise and expand in consciousness. You can tap in anytime, in the physical or non-physical, once you're attuned at that level. That comes with time for most people, although some already have it, or get it quickly.

It's a good thing there's no limit on what I (or anyone who's clear and focused) can do in the non-physical, because in the physical, we can't answer the growing number of email questions we receive, nor give email advice. Coming to the site does tap you into the uplifting field of resonance, and people say they get a lot from that.

To receive inspirational notes, free articles, event announcements, and invitations, join the newsletter list at www.DivineOpenings.com.

Our website, online retreats, conference calls and sessions are designed to support you in your evolution. Visit www.DivineOpenings.com often, read today's quote, peruse the free material, comment on the blog, enjoy the color art in the gallery, and see "what's new." The site is an ever-expanding world, and we keep it fresh for you.

VERY IMPORTANT!

Please read carefully before proceeding:
I am an evolutionary agent of Divine Energy/Light/Intelligence
and I use the words in this book, the art, my music, my intention, and other
direct non-physical means to translate and convey it to you.

EACH TIME YOU come to a work of art in the book and gaze at it with the intention of receiving a Divine Opening, you will. A casual glance will not give a Divine Opening unasked for. The Divine Opening "expands your pipes" and opens you to let in more Grace.

- Wait at least seven days between Divine Openings. More and faster is *not better*, cowboys and cowgirls. Each Divine Opening needs time to integrate and unfold fully before adding new input. In general, slow down everywhere in your life so you can feel more.

- Pregnant women past the second trimester may not receive Divine Openings until after delivery of the baby. Just read the book and allow it to give you Divine Mother Hugs.

- Those with serious mental disorders should receive sessions before doing Divine Openings.

Work with Lola or another Divine Openings Giver in person or by phone. See the directory on our site.

- Alcohol or mood altering drugs of any type interfere with your feeling processes and prevent the full benefit of Divine Openings. Divine Openings can help you stop needing and wanting them, so do your best with this as you begin. Those with active substance addictions may or may not need sessions to help them get off the substance. As an interesting perspective, since Lola's vibration is so high, if she ingests a substance now, it either takes her to a lower vibration, or she feels no difference!

- Divine Openings are for those eighteen years or older. Those under eighteen can receive another form of Opening to help them develop and succeed in life. Contact us.

- Receive only one Divine Opening per week from any source. *"Advanced" people are no exception.* More than that can be too intense, and the point is to enjoy your evolution! It used to be OK to do more, but now the energy is so big, that could be unnecessarily rigorous. *Don't speed up the energy faster than you can release resistance to it.* You can read past a Divine Opening artwork and come back later, but *read the book in order each time you read it.*

- Each Divine Opening experience is different, so don't compare yours to anyone else's, or have any expectations. If you don't feel anything, it means nothing about the power of it. Your mind might argue about this, and just ignore it if it does.

YOU DON'T NEED a Divine Opening every week forever. You'll soon access this Grace state by just intending it. One day you'll come to live in that state of Grace and flow most of the time.

The awakening of Divine Intelligence within you automatically resolves anything it stirs up very quickly if you will relax, dismiss judgment, and allow the feeling to move up. Don't use other modalities to try to relieve or "fix" the after-effects of a Divine Opening—it makes it worse. It also contradicts the intention to feel everything. Don't try to make the feelings (valuable messengers) go away! Resisting lower feelings got you where you are, and embracing them will take you to a realm of self-empowerment beyond your highest expectations. Be with and embrace them softly, sweetly, kindly, and they will move up faster. Most modalities are about making the feelings or the pain go away, but Divine Openings shows you later in this book how to stop creating pain, suffering, and difficulty at the core rather than just relieving the symptoms.

You could benefit from massage, bodywork (*not* energy work!), Rolfing, Feldenkrais, yoga, chiropractic, acupuncture, music, dancing, and exercise to help the slower, denser physical self to relax, let go, and allow the flow.

Next, you will receive a Divine Opening from a work of art. People report that the black and white art in the book works just as well, but some prefer the color artworks in the Art Gallery at www.DivineOpenings.com.

Enjoy. Because it's all about joy.

Divine Opening

Your first Divine Opening is a special occasion that formally initiates you to a new level of enlightenment. Take a moment now to review where you have been in your life, let go of, and say goodbye to the past. You could offer appreciation for the Grace you are about to let in.

Gaze gently at the work of art for about two minutes. Get out of the way.

Simply allow the Divine Grace to do it all.

Then close your eyes, lie down, and rest for fifteen minutes or longer.

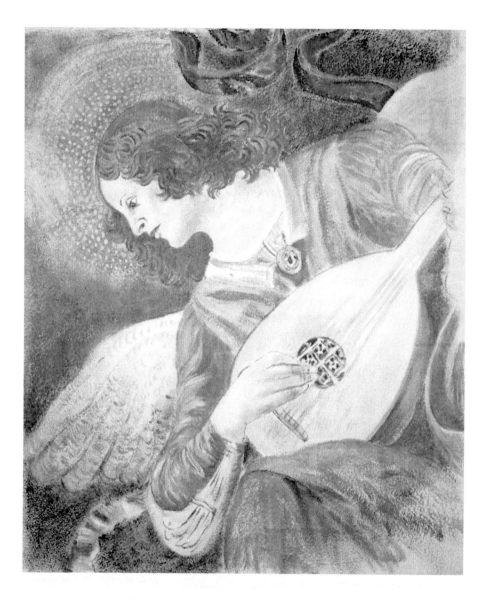

Figure 1—Angel, a five foot mural by Lola Jones,
her interpretation after Italian master Mellozo da Forli's Angel With Lute

After Your First Divine Opening

NOW YOU HAVE had your first Divine Opening, an initiation to enlightenment, or a deepening into the next level. It works on the subtle planes. Regardless of how much or how little you can perceive, *it is working on you just the same, and will continue to for months and years to come.* It is cumulative, and the effect does build with each successive Divine Opening.

You may feel instantly blissful, then in the next few days you may feel some old unwanted emotions or stagnant vibrations moving up. Let it move. Allowing energy and vibration to move up is a key to your freedom. This book guides you through the movement.

Sometimes you feel nothing special, and then remarkable changes start occurring in the following weeks, in your body, mind, and feelings—in your life, and even in the people around you. Take care to notice and appreciate every little wonderful thing that occurs.

Your Large Self designed your experience just for you, so rather than comparing your experience to someone else's or to something you read in a spiritual book or this book, *appreciate your experience.* No two Divine Openings are alike; so don't expect the same one ever again. Let go of each experience, and be open new ones each time—as in Life!

Subtle is just as powerful. Let go of expectations and judgments. While live, in-person, or phone Divine Openings are usually more intense, we hear many dramatic exceptions to that from readers. Some people get full liberation just from this book. Others need or desire more help letting go of resistance.

Please journal to *yourself* about your progress, and let me know your *successes* in *short* emails to celebrate@lolajones.com. I cannot answer all emails, nor counsel people by email, but www.DivineOpenings.com gives you bountiful options for personal or online support.

Each Divine Opening works on you intensely for weeks, months, and years, so notice and appreciate everything that happens in your inner and outer world, even those things you don't understand yet. Your life will forever be affected, made easier, and eventually make more sense.

Coughing Up a Hairball, Hitting A Speed Bump

LET'S COVER THIS now, since you've had your first Divine Opening. You're opening to experience a fuller range of emotions, from profound bliss, to emotions you'd probably label as "unwanted." When you decide to awaken, you're asking Grace to raise your vibration, and as that happens, lower vibrational energies activate and begin to move upward rapidly, often en masse. Maybe in the past you'd get stuck in the lower feelings, but with the Grace-assist of Divine Openings, they move quickly (unless you resist them.) We are deeply brainwashed that we have to learn by suffering, but if you can let go of that, suffering isn't necessary at all. Just feel your feelings and let them move. If you don't try to fix the feeling or *make it go away,* and don't make it wrong, you won't suffer. Resistance turns mere pain into suffering.

I cannot emphasize this enough because when you're caught up in some feeling or situation you might forget that the emotion is perfect. Emotion, and outer things changing, are signs things are moving, so appreciate and value all emotions and events—*all of them!* Lower vibrations are rising, and your old consciousness is actually crumbling. Mountains of energies from decades and eons ago are rising in vibration, en masse.

Those vibrations are not new. They were affecting your reality, whether you knew about them or not. Soon you will welcome and even enjoy all emotions as they arise and rise in vibration. It quickly brings freedom. But for now, you might want some guidance about how to deal with the denser, heavier feelings, which you may (or may not) feel as they move upward to higher feelings.

People are accustomed to taking unwanted emotions too seriously, so I came up with a benign and humorous term to lighten it up: "coughing up a hairball" (like cats do.) One student called it "hitting a speed bump." It encourages people to lighten up about it, and so move through it faster—even to laugh about it and enjoy the movement more. It doesn't have to be heavy unless you resist. Let your mantra be "it all moves easily," and that becomes your reality.

Generally, any unwanted feeling or manifestation could be called a hairball or speed bump, and it does indeed move on quickly if you don't resist, fight, or try to escape it. Fear, anxiety, worry, anger, uncontrollable rage, grief, depression, aggravation, jealousy, illness, fatigue, headache, nausea, digestive upsets, odd physical sensations, odd automatic body movements that you can't control, upsets with others, financial scares, and setbacks—all of these can and do move easily! Those vibrations have needed to move for a long time. The best news is now, if you stop resisting, those old feelings don't have to play out the hardest way, as unwanted events, or conditions, people, or illnesses in your life. The bulk of your density usually lightens in the first few months of Divine Openings, *if you'll let go*. It doesn't go on forever—those old days of endless processing are over.

Full body bliss and lower energies moving up—you'll feel it all. We had a good laugh when a few clients actually felt something physically scratchy in their throats like a hairball! Intend for your awakening to happen with ease, Grace, and humor, and it can. Resist nothing and value and accept all feelings, and your awakening can be smooth. Again, let go of the human belief in the value of suffering. There is *no value in suffering* unless it's the *only way* you'll let yourself evolve.

Declare ease and Grace. I did, and I got it. Some of you actually *need* flash and drama so you know that "something big" is going on. Once your awakening begins, it's on cruise control with Grace driving, so your most joyful option is to let go and let it happen with love and joy instead of lessons and pain. If things in your life break down, you weren't letting it happen any other way. The hard way *does* work eventually, but you can choose the easy way—and this book tells you precisely how.

Let it move with maximum ease, grace, and humor.

Appreciate the Larger non-physical aspect of you for helping you move those dense old postures, masks, strategies, defenses, structures, and patterns that you had unconsciously created through the years. They were embedded down to the cells and atoms. All you need do is open to experience, and fully feel all those energies as they rise in vibration, literally making you lighter, brighter, more radiant. Each Divine Opening pre-programs the emergence and eventual dissolution of old energies, patterns, and habits that no longer serve you. It points up the old small-self density that is not you, the fearful illusion and pain your mind created, and it all rises in vibration as it is fully felt. Again: if you don't resist it, pain doesn't become suffering. Big difference. Experiencing it without resistance means without running from it, complaining, analyzing, talking about it, or acting it out. Just feel it softly, gently, with compassion for yourself. Any emotion, experienced fully, alchemically rises to a higher vibration.

I'll remind you repeatedly, because at first, when we feel an unwanted emotion, our old conditioned response is to make it wrong. It is perfect. It must move up to allow change. If you continue to struggle, avoid, or resist lower feelings, get the "Dive In And Be With It" audio set that gently walks you through it. My voice sets up a powerful vortex that accelerates your progress, and helps train you to tune into that by yourself. Find it at www.DivineOpenings.com.

Any emotion fully experienced moves up into a higher vibration.

Humans call some emotions negative and some positive, but it's all valuable information. Now, don't go digging for negativity! That delays enlightenment. You actually create negativity by looking for it, and it never ends (have you noticed that?) With Divine Openings, Life presents to you anything you need to deal with, in perfect timing. Live life and be happy, and feelings, events, or circumstances that need to move will arise as needed in the course of living. *Let go of the old paradigm* of clearing, healing, and learning lessons. "Working" on spiritual and personal growth is addictively ingrained in many well-meaning people. If you keep working on yourself, you're choosing to live in the old paradigm, and it's a tough reality. As soon as you decide your life is about joy rather than "learning lessons" it gets really good. Evolution just *happens* with Divine Openings.

Anytime something happens that isn't what you want, or you feel something you don't like, it's just life telling you, "Here's a place where you're out of alignment with your Large Self, so it hurts." "Here's a place where you're not being your true self, so it's painful." "Here's an opportunity to let go and let The Divine open you up." You'll soon know how to do this, and it is not work.

When something arises after a Divine Opening (or anytime from now on) and it doesn't feel good, thoroughly experience it (feel it without the mental story about it—with no words) and it will move up to a higher vibration. Later in the book we give you a Diving In process to help you, but Divine Openings pre-programs it to move up naturally if you relax and soften—there is no work to do, no analyzing, and no "processing." Most modalities keep you on the old fix-it hamster wheel, and worse, keep you dependent on others. Go within and stop seeking answers "out there." Commit to take every feeling, every problem, and every joy to The Presence within first.

Something might occur, like a problem at work. Just experience the pure feeling. If something makes you sad, experience the sadness. If you get fearful, feel the fear, and it too will move up.

In other words, experience it all internally. Don't think about it, analyze it, tell yourself the story, or talk about it to others. Feel it. If you can relax and let it flow through you it quickly passes. Where we get stuck is in the drama of retelling the "story," judging the situation or person, thinking how wrong or unfair it is. The story perpetuates the feeling and generates more of it. Stay out of the story and just experience life as it is. As enlightenment unfolds, you value being happy and loving more than being right about your story. You ignore your disempowering stories.

After a Divine Opening you may get depressed, angry, enraged, or sad for no reason. Just be with it and observe it, saying to yourself, "Oh, I'm depressed," or "Oh, I'm sad." There is nothing to do, and if you can, don't say anything about it to anyone else. Take it within to The Presence.

Though it feels like it's happening right now, it's usually not—it's actually old energy.

Once you can experience your emotions internally instead of playing them out externally your life becomes a drama-free zone. The help from Grace makes it possible with much more ease. I think back on times when I tried to stay out of conflicts with my ex and could not do it. Now it seems inconceivable to live in that kind of drama, and I laugh to myself, "What was I thinking?" But that was a different consciousness, and in this new consciousness, you'll find that so many of the old problems just don't exist anymore, and it seems odd you ever had them.

For example, most conflicts and unhappiness with other people diminish to nothing once you realize how you created those relationships. People begin to act completely differently with you at a certain stage of your awakening. Typically the changes fall into three categories: 1.) They shift. 2.) Your perception shifts and you're no longer bothered by it. 3.) You part easily.

Your greatest power lies in cleaning up your own emotions before speaking to someone or acting on it. There are plenty of processes later on in the book to help you do that.

Try not to speak to anyone or make important decisions while you're in lower emotional states. Even if it seems like they are doing something to you or that you must act, see if you can wait until you're clear. It may look like the cause of the emotion is "out there," but stay focused within, where your power is, as much as you can. This becomes your powerful new habit.

Once you've experienced your own emotions fully, thus reclaimed that tied up emotional energy, you have a clearer, brighter view of the situation. If you still need to say something to the other person, your words are clean and effective; your actions are powerful and constructive. They can hear you, perhaps for the first time, and your relationship improves. I'll say it again later:

Negative emotion is for "internal use only."

Once you're clear, you speak from your Large Self without blame, with no emotional charge nor a trace of victimhood. From an innocent and pure place, you might tell someone how you feel or felt, or what you want. You usually won't need to, though, because when "you are there for you emotionally," others naturally join you. Once you're out of negative emotion you communicate better. But if you blow up and vent on someone, you are human. Just take responsibility, tell them you should have taken it within instead of taking it out on them, and you are back in integrity. They will respect you for that.

Once a relative criticized me in front of a friend, telling him all of my faults from her perspective. After going to bed, I felt through it thoroughly, without trying to fix it. The next morning I was centered and in my heart, and I knew I could communicate well. When my friend left the room, I gave the relative a hug, and tears came to my eyes -- not the tears of a victim or a blamer, but the tears of an open heart. I thought of how I could make it more about "how I feel" than about "what she did." So I said, "It hurts when you say things like that about me, especially to others." She immediately apologized and I just listened as she talked about her unhappiness. She was very depressed about her husband's disability since his stroke. Our relationship moved up to yet a new level.

There are times when you will use raw anger constructively to make a difference, to move yourself up from depression, fear, grief or despair to stand up to someone, help someone you love, or change a situation. Anger is powerful when used consciously and selectively—when you are its master rather than taken over by it unconsciously. You'll receive all the processes you need to help you put this into practice in the real world.

Why there is so much emphasis on emotion in Divine Openings:

- Emotions are your Instrument Panel indicator of where you are, and which way to go. You'll learn and experience this in detail throughout this book. Too many people develop high spiritual knowledge, but their practical life still doesn't work well. Learning to take accurate Instrument Panel readings helps life make more sense and work out better.

- Experiences, bodily conditions, finances and relationships all reflect the emotional energy you're radiating. Once you master emotion *you can manifest powerfully.* When you can move emotional energy, you can move any energy. Manifesting is literally the ability to focus and flow energy.

- Emotional mastery is prerequisite to enlightenment. No amount of esoteric knowledge can substitute. It's possible to have flashes of profound illumination *but lose it* when confronted with emotional or challenging life situations. Paradoxically, when you can be with any feeling, you will feel good most of the time, and it helps sustain your enlightenment.

Being With What Is

IN ORDER TO GAIN this ability to give Divine Grace, I spent twenty-one days in an austere silent process in India communing only with God within. Going to India isn't necessary—that's just how I happened to do it, and it was perfect for me. Now I initiate people anywhere. It was so delicious that I scarcely noticed the hard concrete floors we sat on, the tiny army beds in dorm rooms with sixteen other women, and the awful food. Two hundred fifty other people from around the world were there, but I didn't get to know any of them until it was over. My focus was inward—I wasn't there to socialize—I was there to go within and end my outer dependence. While not all observed strict silence, I did. No speaking and only enough eye contact to avoid bumping into people in the dorm hallways. The silence was profoundly and permanently transformative for me.

In that sheltered, secluded environment, we had nothing else to do or attend to. I chose not to communicate with home by phone or email except on a couple of occasions when I emailed briefly to say I was alive and well. My fervent aim was to go within without distraction, and commune only with The Presence. I embraced the opportunity fully, and it changed my life.

What a deep respite it was—perhaps a once-in-a-lifetime opportunity to have three weeks to do nothing but commune with The Divine. It was Heaven! It left me more relaxed than I'd ever been in my entire life. And it has lasted in spite of the much busier schedule that I now have since the success of Divine Openings, with many projects, events, courses, music, and art being produced.

The chronic tension and anxiety I carried my whole life disappeared permanently. If I get stressed, I notice it, relax and breathe, and it leaves, because my body is awake and alive with Divine consciousness. It corrects itself with just a little awareness, or with a little nudge from body-work or exercise. Energy work is unnecessary once you learn how to manage your own energy.

Emotions of every kind rippled through me one after the other during the twenty-one days of silence. First, terror when my passport was taken away to a nearby town to be photocopied. The efficiency level of the people I had encountered on my journey to the campus had not given me any confidence that I'd ever see my passport again. I lay awake terrified all night the first night certain I'd be stranded in India if they lost it, but I sensed this drama merely put the spotlight on decades of old fears. It was an invitation for me to experience the fear fully, without trying to fix it or make it go away, and so reclaim that energy and raise the vibration of it.

Any feeling we're willing to be with and experience fully rises in vibration, then that energy becomes available for constructive uses. By the second day the fear was bearable, by the third day it was a non-issue, and I actually laughed as my passport was handed back to me on the fourth day, long after they had said I'd get it back. I learned that when a person fully embraces one or two core emotions, and truly experiences them to the depths, not only do they rise in frequency, all emotions are soon mastered. You don't have to wade individually through every emotion, vibration, and trauma you've ever experienced in your history, thank God. Those old days of handling issues one at a time, and layer after layer, *are over.* You will experience en masse resolution and evolution. You're being prepared for the processes later in the book. Go slowly! If you feel a need to skip ahead or rush, that's your mind interfering. *Slow down, savor, and lay a solid foundation.*

Emotion came in waves, flowing through me and the others, often without reason. Causeless joy, causeless anger, sadness without content. Tears came and left again just as suddenly. So much of what we feel is not even ours. We pick it up from Ancient Mind, a massive and powerful collective thought form. We pick up Ancient Mind's vibrations and think it is ours. Then we attract more of whatever we focus upon, and on it goes, down through the generations. Every thought that has ever been thought is still accessible.

Waves of angst crashed over me as I waded into a sea of inner questions, doubts, sadness and grief. I had been in a steady, happy place back at home. I so clearly knew the importance of feeling good. When I felt all those strong emotions, I wondered, "What am I doing here? I feel so much worse than before I came!" Yet there were some key things in my life that were still stuck after many years on the path and I knew deep down I was in the right place. There were obviously blind spots I was not aware of holding me back. I'd not been able to even identify them, much less change them. Somehow I knew the silence would give me the total freedom I sought. It did, and it has lasted.

The Ancient Mind has long held all but a few enlightened beings in a drama of survival and lack—stuck in suffering, disempowerment and separation from the flow of Life. But fortunately Grace does for us that we cannot do for ourselves. Every very powerful agent of The Divine that has walked the planet came to give us a gift of Grace—to lift us up in ways that our own human efforts simply couldn't do.

Surprisingly, the emotion I struggled with longer than anything else was anger at those people who could not be quiet, who whispered with the other people in our dorm room and in the dining hall, disturbing our delicious sacred silence. I knew they were terrified of the silence and of facing themselves in it, but I wanted them to be quiet and let *me* enjoy it. And how dare they break the rules! This indignation was odd; I'm not a rule follower myself. I wrestled with my harsh judgment of them longest and hardest of all, while the "big" life issues shifted with total ease!

Judgment is a deeply ingrained human habit. Many religions are even built on it. Finally I could just be present with my judgment, and let it be. "So I'm judging them as weak and inconsiderate because they're wasting their precious time here. So be it!" Then it dissolved and I looked at them with compassion. Voila!

As each wave of every imaginable emotion passed, I felt steadily more able to stand in them unfazed, increasingly washed and opened, and eventually felt more and more wonderful. A new hope began to sprout in the hard, parched ground of my many years of endless seeking and growing discouragement. This was different than anything before it. I felt a depth and a certainty within myself begin to open up. My greatest desire was to become totally inner directed, free of the need to go to others for answers and healing—to have my own main line to The Divine. In the deep, rich, increasingly thought-free silence, that wish was coming true.

After much letting go, I began to move from hope to joy to ecstasy, with the occasional dip into feelings we call negative, then I began to accept and welcome even those feelings—watching myself experience them without identifying them as me, and without labeling them as good or bad. They all became "just temporary experiences," and they all passed. Equanimity and acceptance of all feelings replaced the rollercoaster ride I'd been on my entire life—a ride I thought I was stuck with. Equanimity is, quite simply, being OK with what is.

Although a few days were intensely difficult, overall it was one of the most beautiful, awe-inspiring and precious twenty-one days of my life. A few minutes of bitter tears, an hour of deep pain, or a day of anger was always followed by profound peace or even bliss. As any vibration is fully experienced and not run from, it always rises into higher and finer vibration, leaving only our natural, unadulterated Large Self. Those feelings weren't me! How fascinating to experience it firsthand, while cradled securely in the arms of The Divine.

I relaxed further once I saw the possibilities. It always resolved anything it brought up with such beauty and simplicity. As long as I didn't resist, I was free, no matter how I was feeling. Fear of feeling and resistance to feeling causes more suffering than the original feeling itself. I saw other people resisting and not getting this, and yes they did suffer. Those who resisted hard, about eighty percent of the people, got physically ill. I didn't resist the feelings, didn't get sick, and never again would be afraid of any feeling. This resulted in a remarkable, lasting freedom.

Back at home I was soon able to be as centered, productive, and "OK" while feeling grief as while feeling ecstasy, whereas before, a strong negative feeling would almost certainly derail my productivity and happiness that day, or even for months or years at a time. There was now a certainty deep within me that popping back up to happiness was natural—a certainty that anything except happiness was merely a *temporary* separation from my Large Self. All I had to do was relax and let go, embrace and dive into the feeling, to return gently to my Large Self (much more on precisely how to do this comes later in the book.)

Within a few months of the delicious twenty-one days I was, for the first time in my life, no longer at the effect of outside circumstances, other people, negative emotions, the world, the economy, or the dense vibrations of the Ancient Mind. My center was solid; I was grounded like a rock. Nothing brought me down for long. I felt light, transparent, and unsinkable.

Be with what is and you are free.

Energy And Emotion Must Move

EMOTION AND ENERGY are supposed to move and flow through us. When emotion or energy is resisted and can't move, we get out of sync with the Flow of Life. Every disease or malady can be traced back to energy that was not allowed to move freely.

Too many spiritual people try to avoid lower emotions, magically transcend them, make them go away with sessions or modalities, or deny them. They want to avoid any "bad" lower emotions and leap straight up into higher ones. I call that a "spiritual bypass." Interestingly, spiritual development is stunted until you deal with the very human realm of emotions. Enlightenment requires fully embracing the whole human experience, fully embodying in the physical—not rising above it or escaping it. As enlightened humans, we're bringing Heaven to Earth, not looking for a fast pass out of here.

When we try to push negative feelings away they last longer, because by focusing on what we don't want, we give them more life and energy. When we try to cling to positive feelings or experiences, we're operating as if there is a scarcity of them. When we realize that there is an endless supply there is no need to try to freeze them and keep them. Let them flow. Stop trying to hold onto positive emotions or experiences, or trying to push away negative emotions or experiences, since doing either is trying to stop something that is innately designed to flow.

It's your birthday party and you open a fabulous gift: you savor it, you pass it around and enjoy it as long as you can, but the next gift you open will be different. It won't be the same as that one, but you can enjoy the next one too, and then move on to the next gift, and the next. Experiences are like that. Blissful or painful they come and go, and there will be more. Source provides an endless supply of delights and experiences, and when we're open and relaxed, each one gets sweeter than the last, eternally.

Don't hold onto the gift.
Hold onto The Giver.

Assisted by the initiations we received from our monk-like guides, I was soon able to "be with" and allow any negative thought or emotion to move on through me within minutes of its arising, no matter how heavy, how old, or how strong. Eventually everything I felt or thought gently passed, leaving at the very least peace, emptiness, and a quiet, still mind in its wake, and at the very best, bliss. It was hugely freeing.

As resistance to "what is" relaxed, all my senses opened up, and I began to feel things with a new intensity. Even my sense of smell improved. I felt wide open and wide-eyed, like a new baby. Now I can take an emotion that used to sink me for months or years and dive so deeply into it, embrace it softly and feel it fully, while sitting with my eyes closed (or even while going about my day) that it literally explodes into multi-colored bliss inside me within minutes. At the bottom of everything is bliss. At my core is bliss. This is no surprise once you realize that your Large Self experiences only bliss. When you're experiencing something less, you're just not fully in alignment with your Large Self. You've wandered off course and gotten separated from the Oneness, the Flow of Life. Soon you'll know how to get back home easily.

You will soon be able to easily observe yourself "having" emotions without getting mired "in" them. Nothing will ever be as gripping as it used to be. Clients tell me this all the time. Nothing bothers them as much anymore. I feel everything, but I cannot imagine ever being terribly devastated again by anything. Later on in the book, you'll receive a process called Diving In that helps you master this.

Life may be terminal, but it's certainly not that serious.

What I do now, for others and myself, is beyond healing, cleansing, clearing, energy work or therapy. It affects the vibration permanently; whereas energy work just adjusts something that people usually soon recreate the way it was, because the habits that generated that vibration haven't changed. Divine Openings awakens people with pure Energy/Light/Intelligence. The planet, the sun, the Internet, computers, money, thought, rocks, the ocean, and you and me are made of Energy/Light/Intelligence, but many humans have let their frequency get distorted. As you awaken and vibrate with a pure, undistorted frequency that's in alignment with the Flow of Life, issues and problems disappear naturally, because they don't resonate with you anymore.

What's most real is invisible and can't be seen. Manifest physical reality is made of subtle non-stuff few can see. Scientists have been dropping clues for us for at least fifty years. They know that nothing is solid—what they can't explain is why it acts and appears solid to us. What physicists have found is so fantastically surreal; most of them quickly turn a blind eye to how wild it is. They "forget" what they saw, because the mind has difficulty grasping it.

The birth of everything is in the non-physical. We're remembering that, and putting more attention and focus on creating in the non-physical rather than working so hard on the physical level—the hardest, densest level at which to work. Each time this awareness drops more deeply into your knowing you become free of the illusion of anything being solid or unchangeable. Everything is born of pure possibility. Millions of years ago, you were just a possibility.

Worthiness

YOU EXIST. You were given life. Therefore you are worthy. Period. End of subject. You're part of the All That Is, so you're worthy. You have possibly been working too hard to attain something you already have, or to prove something that was never in question—your worth. Unworthiness is a mind-construct. Unworthiness doesn't really exist. Even people you think of as bad or evil are worthy, as The Divine gave them life and Free Will to do anything they chose. Yes, Hitler went back to pure positive energy, or Heaven, just like Mother Teresa. The Indweller does not judge what you choose to do with your gift of Life, but gives Free Will to all, knowing there is no ultimate risk for an eternal being. Mistakes don't exist either, and are not tallied by The Divine nor held against you. Karma is a primitive religious concept, much like Hell. They both deny Grace, and you can let go of them now. Each life, each day, each moment, is a fresh new start.

Life is about joy and love—if you'll allow it. We are here to live, laugh, love, enjoy, create, expand and choose whatever we want. There is nothing to earn, get, overcome, or prove. Many people concluded that they were not good enough, or that if they had been worthy, they would have gotten the love and care they wanted, the popularity, or the good stuff. It had nothing to do with worthiness. We have mistakenly transferred human qualities onto God. For example, when our parents or other humans judged us instead of loving us unconditionally, we concluded that God is the same way. Human love is fickle and conditional. Divine Love is unfailing and unconditional. God, your Large Self, adores you no matter what.

Religions sometimes tell us we are unworthy. If you believe it's true you will live the consequences of that belief. Our beliefs play out in our reality, making them seem all the more real because "proof" always shows up to match our beliefs.

You learned unworthiness from other people who were separated from their Large Selves. They "proved" that belief over and over, and you bought it. You took on vibrations from them in order to be like them, and so fit in and be safe. This happened so long ago that you don't remember doing it. If you've never felt anything else, you are accustomed to it, and you don't question it. And you can't feel how damaging it is. If it feels bad, it's not your Divine state. If it feels bad, that tells you you're out of alignment with what God thinks about it. Unworthiness feels bad, and it should, because it indicates your separation from God *on that subject*. The Divine loves you, and when you disagree and say you are unworthy, you are out of alignment with The Very One who created you. Know your worthiness and let in the unlimited good that flows to you constantly.

Feelings of unworthiness are one of the biggest blocks to receiving Divine Grace, so the sooner you can release those judgments against yourself, the more fully you can receive the good that is flowing to you and through you all the time. Unworthiness is a lie and a mistake. Let it go. Decide you are worthy right now! God already has. Why not agree and get back in alignment with The All That Is?

Worthiness is a given. You may let in all the good now.

The four most common resistances that slow down one's liberation are:
1) Unworthiness—You don't let the good in if you don't believe you're worthy of it.
Accept your worthiness now. This book will help you realize your worthiness.
2) Addictions—They usurp your will, use your power, and skew your choices. Release them.
3) Love that's not flowing with all people in your life, current and past—We address this later.
4) A very strong, over-dominant left brain—Let me sing to your soul, because you'll never, ever get Divine Openings with your brain. It just isn't capable of containing or explaining it.

It's your life and you're important.
Prioritize yourself.

What Is Compassion?

IF SOMEONE YOU LOVE fell into a deep well filled with water, with no way to climb out, what would you do? Would you jump in out of sympathy? If you did, what good would you do? What you'd probably decide to do is get a rope and stay up there in safety while pulling them out. It's the same with any deep dark emotional, spiritual, mental or physical hole that your friend or family member, community member, or nation finds itself in. Descending to that low feeling place doesn't help anyone out of it. It lowers your ability to be of any service to anyone.

In this process, focus on yourself for now. You can help others when you are liberated.

We got stuck with the odd idea that compassion is the same as commiserating, or sharing the burden. This has become so pervasive that people expect you to grieve with them, suffer with them, lament, and feel down with them. If you stay up, you are of more service to everyone, especially yourself. When someone is suffering, you can hear them and let them know you hear them, but don't go down there to that low place with them. Stay "up" no matter what is going on around you.

Compassion for your self is primary. Before you read on, make a decision to be easy on yourself. Many spiritual people have compassion for everyone—except themselves. Make peace with wherever you are right this minute, knowing you did the best you could, and that now you are moving forward, not looking back. Making peace with who you are and where you are frees you to enjoy life on your journey, right now, today, just as you are. You are where you are! God is not judging—why are you? Are you as compassionate to yourself as you are to others?

Whatever you experience in this process is perfect. You are never really stuck. Just keep going. Give yourself lots of encouragement and support in this and in every area of your life. As the very entertaining Cajun minister Jesse DuPlantis said, "If you're going through Hell, don't stop! Keep moving!"

Your Past Was Leading You To NOW

I AM *NOT* SAYING all the spiritual stuff you learned in this lifetime before you came to Divine Openings was necessary to help you "get" Divine Openings. *It was not necessary.* Beginners often get it *faster* because they're empty and uncluttered to start with. Previous study is often a handicap, because the mind is full of old stuff that didn't end your seeking. I mean in the larger sense of human evolution you've been leading up to this place and time for eons, despite the detours.

Life Force spent billions of years evolving this environment for You. Then it evolved You. You continue to evolve You, and will for eternity. Source loves to create and expand, and never stops. There is no end destination. This in itself is a freeing notion. You will never be done, so you can stop being concerned with perfection, completion, being behind, or "getting to enlightenment." Enjoy this moment as if it is Christmas Eve and you are about to open the most astounding pile of presents you have ever received. Isn't that a good feeling?

This moment is all there really is. This book is about being happy in this moment, and when you are happy in this moment, you are in agreement with The Presence. The time for enlightenment is NOW. The time for mankind to wake up is NOW. The methods are right here for you, right NOW, in this book. You are NOW on your way to enlightenment. Really! Finally.

Savor the journey. It's been a long time coming. On my spiritual path, for decades it seemed it would never come, but it's here. It requires little from you, because by Grace it is given to you. Universal Intelligence is intervening and giving it to you where you were not able to find it or figure it out from limited human intelligence.

It has always been that way. Monks would fervently study, pray and give devotions and service for years with no sign of enlightenment, and then one day, if they were fortunate, Grace opened them up instantly out of the blue. Divine Openings opens you to let it in.

One thing was certain—once my awakening began, life was never mundane again.

This moment is a new beginning, and eternity is full of endless new beginnings.

Many Personalities

YOU WILL DISCOVER you are not one single personality. You are many. Just observe them as they come and go in response to circumstances. At various times, for example, you might be the taskmaster, the loafer, the child, the priest, the hedonist, the fearful one, the miser, the leader, the follower, the dreamer, the lover, the nurturer, or the artist. Resisting the unwanted aspects of yourself only strengthens them. What you resist persists. Just watch them come and go, observe, judge not, and embrace them all. That awareness is all you need. Over time, you will become more your authentic core self. Just as you flow emotions, flow through these personalities. Don't get caught up in fixing or processing them. That's playing their game, you'll never win, and it will never end. Let them come and go without resistance and they move on, as all energy wants to do.

There may even be times that you loathe yourself as you feel aspects of you that are far separated from your Divinity. You may feel embarrassed, guilty, shamed, or disgusted by things you've said or done. Be with those feelings, and drop the story about what you did. Feel with no words. Just feel. Really, that's all you need to do. The Presence is not judging you, so feel the feelings and drop the story. Once the feelings move, your vibration rises, which puts you in alignment with The Presence, who adores you, no matter what. Grace helps you feel those unwanted contrasts and then you know more clearly what you do want.

Again, I never talk about ego. The ego is an artificial construct that doesn't really exist, and struggling with any illusion is insane. What you resist persists. You need a sense of separate self to ensure your survival in the physical plane. People with what are labeled "big egos" are responsible for some of the most beneficial discoveries and events in history. Don't make it wrong, and don't worry about it. Just focus on being your Large Self, and you'll have no need to be concerned with ego. Your small self naturally refines itself as you unfold. Your small self may go through stages, from "I'm worthless" to "I'm better than everyone" to a more mature appreciation of *your authentic magnificence.* You see, once again, there is no "work" to do. Letting go of processing and working on one's self is often exactly like breaking an addiction. Just stop working on yourself and live.

Keep It Simple For Best Results

NO ONE LIKES to be told what to do, and that's natural. *Do whatever you please,* yet if you want to be one of those people who gets the big results, let go of everything. Even if something once served you, if it had been working all that well, you simply wouldn't be here, still seeking. Divine Openings brings unimaginable freedom when you keep it simple.

For three years I dropped everything spiritual except Divine Openings. It gave me tremendous inner power, and finally ended my dependence on other people and outer stuff. When we seek, ask, and grasp outside (which I did for twenty-five years) awakening is *impossible.* Our own guidance is heard only when we stop drowning it out with too many other voices and inputs. Your Large Self can get in the driver's seat only if you make empty space for it there. Since my twenty-one glorious days of cold-turkey, no-seeking, let-it-all-go, I'm-finally-here silence, I am not interested in spiritual books, metaphysical events, or seminars. I'd do those things if I felt like it, but that stuff is incredibly boring to me now. If I read something inspirational occasionally, it's for the simple enjoyment of it. Mostly I read upbeat fiction and humor.

Most (not all) spiritual books, therapy, seminars, readings, energy work, and emotional/spiritual "healing" modalities are contradictory to Divine Openings. That's going to become clearer to you as you go; just ponder this for now. We don't want to balance your energy for you, clear negativity for you, or fix or heal you; we give you the power and show you how do it for yourself, anytime, anywhere. The reason energy work makes people feel better temporarily, but isn't lasting, is they go back to the same vibrational habits and create the same conditions over again. Moreover, by believing there's something to clear or heal, they continually create things to go get cleared or healed, and it *never ends.* It's a treadmill.

Divine Openings isn't "energy work," nor is it any type of "work." There is no piecemeal tackling of endless issues. You can be *done* with that, although your entire being will evolve, automatically, at a Grace-accelerated rate, directed by the Organizing Intelligence Of Life, eternally.

Use the word "healing" only if you're physically ill. If you're not ill you don't need "healing work"—you only need to wake up. Neither you nor the planet needs "healing." Sorry, but all that is New Age garbage that keeps you on the "there's something wrong with you and the world and you've got to fix it" hamster wheel. Be a powerful creator, not a fixer. Once free, you never have to go back, unless you choose to go back to sleep, or back to seeking (it's the same thing.)

Continue your exercise, yoga, bodywork, and massage. Simple meditations for pleasure are great—drop the complicated ones—it's too much work. Practice your religion if it still speaks to you. You may read and listen to select inspirational things, but if it's contradictory (has you "working on yourself," getting fixed by someone else, "healing your emotions or spirit" (which are not sick and never were!), that's trying to do two opposite things. Get really clear on your choice: awakening, or endless seeking/fixing/working on yourself. *Struggle with and resist the simplicity of this for a while if you need to.* Dive into the feelings it evokes. It's best if you get the "aha" for yourself.

I'll never ask you to have faith or trust. You don't need any. Divine Openings works—if you really do it you'll get proof, and *you only need faith when you have no proof.* If you don't commit and stick with it, you're likely to create "proof" that it doesn't work.

You'll go within in a whole new, very simple way. You'll begin to experience natural, accelerated, joyful evolution. Divine Openings really does free you from suffering, struggle, and having to work on yourself—forever.

YOUR SECOND Divine Opening: You don't have to relate to nor deify this Thai Buddha to get the benefit. I've never studied Buddhism or any such thing (I've never been a "path follower".) The painting just flowed out of my paintbrush after looking at a statue of a Thai Buddha during a road trip. This piece was painted outdoors on a picnic table in a California RV park. Each Divine Opening is unique and won't be like your last. You don't have to feel anything during any Divine Opening for it to work powerfully. Don't work or try. Just open to Divine Grace, and let go.

Divine Opening

This work of art creates a vortex charged with Grace.
Sit quietly and contemplate the image for two minutes.
Then close your eyes and lie down and feel
for at least fifteen or more minutes.

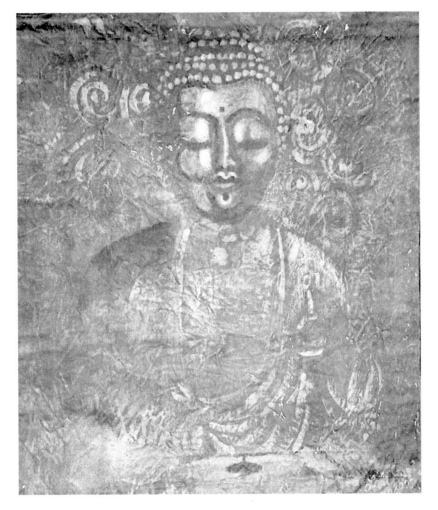

Figure 2—Thai Buddha, a painting by Lola Jones.

Who Is The Divine Presence?

THIS IS NOT a religious book. Anyone with an open mind, of any faith, or no faith at all, will benefit from reading it and from the awakening they receive from it. Although I use terms like The Divine, you can substitute Universal Intelligence, the Organizing Intelligence, The Indweller, Source Energy, The Creator, The Presence, The Light, Jesus, Buddha, Mohammed, Quan Yin, The Mother, Gaia, Nature, Life Force, It, The "I Don't Know What It Is," Fred, or any term you like.

It doesn't matter what you call it, it knows exactly who it is! And you will experience it for yourself in this process rather than taking my word or anyone else's word about it. That said, I will share my perceptions, which are of course filtered through my current state of consciousness and are the highest vibration I had access to when I wrote this. It keeps evolving, and the newest Energy/Light/Intelligence downloads I get go into the online retreat courses, Level 1, 2, and Jumping The Matrix at www.DivineOpenings.com. They go far beyond this book.

Will we ever know the full extent of The Divine Mystery while we are in these bodies, using this brain? Will we define it with words and scientifically nail it down? I doubt it. You'll have plenty of opportunity to know that mystery fully again after this life, when you return to the vast unlimited being you were before this life. Forgetting who we are and remembering it again is a popular game here. Enjoy the unfolding of remembering; the game of hide and seek.

A physician who professed no belief in God took a live course series with me. Atheists don't usually come to me, and I was curious to find out what she would experience. Her eyes lit up and began to shine after her very first Divine Opening—the Presence in her was waking up very fast. It was funny; she had no context for her experience, and it confused her. Something was happening. There was something inside her that she had not believed was there, yet there it was. She had no label or explanation for it. She looked stunned. She darted in and out of class without saying anything, until later, when she'd email me of the changes in her life. In some ways, she's blessed. She can have a direct experience of The Divine without the baggage of cultural conditioning, religion, and dogma.

Her pervasive anxiety about life, relationship, career, and single motherhood disappeared after the first class. Gone. That too can be a bit disorienting for people. When a feeling they've felt their whole lives is gone, it may feel like a void, or even a loss. But it's soon filled with something better.

Whether you believe in it or not, it's already there, and you will experience it. "Experienced" and "advanced" people, the more you let go of all preconceived notions, the more purely you can experience The Presence directly rather than through tired old concepts and filters.

With Divine Openings, we experience a very personal God directly, and most of us lose interest in talking about it, preferring instead to just be in it. Definitions shrink it. People often say to me after a Divine Opening, "It's difficult to explain." I can only smile and nod.

The Creator apparently has levels of being, from the most infinite and large aspect that is indefinable and unknowable to us, down to the most personal aspect that has descended into materiality as us. That largest aspect is impersonal, and frankly, I don't think it is concerned with us; the universe on that scale goes on with or without us. Nobody misses the dinosaurs. It is the more personal, relatable aspect of God that we're concerned with in this book.

The Divine Presence, or our Large Self, is always in bliss, and has no judgments about any of our experiences. The Divine knows its (and our) eternal nature, so death, destruction, our wrongs, errors, and seeming tragedies are flickers on the eternal screen of life. The Presence within us hums along at its high, fine vibration no matter what is going on in our mundane and very human lives. Whether we humans awaken or not, and no matter how our lives go, from its high vibration, the Essence Of Life enjoys living through us. God never dips down into the lower vibrations as we do, no matter what happens. God always sees infinite possibilities, offers solutions, and holds the vibration of bliss for us as a steady homing signal. We came here knowing we would be able to experience lower vibrations and choose among contrasts, or dualities: joy or suffering, enthusiasm or despair, good feelings or bad. Those greater contrasts and choices are a part of the adventure and variety that we deliberately came here to experience. We have free-will choices here. If it seems like you can't yet consciously choose among the contrasts, stick with it and you will get it.

There is much more to you than you see, yet it's not always so easy for you to be sure of that, since you use your physical senses to decide what's real, and your physical senses cannot always perceive the non-physical you. But your Large Self—that vast, unlimited, non-physical aspect of you of which you are but a small physical aspect—is always there for you.

Many of you reading this book already accept that you have lived before this, that there was something before this physical experience, and will be after. But the good news is that you don't have to die and go back to the non-physical to experience that broader non-physical aspect of you; that you have access to it right now and that there is wondrous guidance that is available to you through this inner you that has the full view of reality at all times—a Larger perspective from your Larger Self.

A client sitting in my beautiful living room saw my obviously inspired painting of a Thai goddess (you'll see it later in this book.) She asked if I had past lives in the East. Sure, that goddess was me, but all that I became in past lives is here with me now and becomes even more expanded each day without "doing anything." I don't go back in time to seek or discover anything. As I teach, she smiles, but her energy and wisdom and more are within me here and now. I don't plan sessions or seminars. It comes through in the moment as I relax, let go, and flow.

Your Large Self calls to you to wake up and remember all that *you* are—to experience life as your Large Self does, wise, joyful, with acceptance and compassion, without judgment, without suffering, without struggle. Your Large Self emits a constant homing signal, calling you to live powerfully, magnificently as The Presence in physical form. It's not "healing," it's "waking up."

We eternal beings are never finished, and The Creator is never finished; we're expanding and experimenting. The Creator creates, and co-creating with it, we get to amend, adjust, and improve it to our liking. I was deeply honored when I saw my place in creation—at the center of the Universe. Of course, wondrously, everyone else is also at the center of this holographic Universe.

To fully experience physicality, the formless, non-physical Essence Of Life needs you. When you walk this earth fully awake as your Large Self, knowing that you are a physical point of focus of The Divine, The Creator's desire to play full out in material form is fulfilled. You trek into new frontiers, and create things that have never before been.

The Divine can't do it without you!

People talk about finding their purpose, as if it's some serious, weighty thing. It is such a Puritan ethic to think God has some big heavy expectation of you, or that you have some mission to complete. Nothing could be a bigger distortion of the truth. Your purpose is to enjoy your life! Discover and let go to who you really are—your Large Self, a joyful being—and your talents will multiply and expand without trying. Purpose is a silly New Age notion. Ask a giraffe what its purpose is. Its purpose is to live. I guarantee messages from your guides saying you must fulfill some heavy mission are filtered through some old concept of a God who is demanding of sacrifice and hard work. You are the hands, voice and body of The Divine, but don't get too serious about it. Love, live and enjoy. Serve if it really feels good to you. Playing actually adds just as much value to the planet as work does.

Our Teachers, Ourselves

MY FIRST INITIATION from my first teacher, Maharaji, an enlightened master, happened in 1985. When his own five-year-old son asked him "Who is God?" his answer was, "You can go inside and find out for yourself." He wanted his son to have an original experience, not a hand-me-down concept, even from a master! Maharaji often said, "When you're thirsty, you don't want to talk about water. You don't want a picture of water—you want a drink of water." Maharaji was an international being, and never used Indian terms or practices. He taught us to go directly to God, shed concepts and not depend on the teacher too much. That served me well. I was deeply graced by his meditation process, then I wanted much faster improvement in my outer, practical life, so I moved on after a decade.

A few people will not be able to hear what I'm saying. They might say it didn't help them, or they might get angry at me. When feelings begin to move some run like hell. A few years before encountering Divine Openings and me, one friend of mine had quite a flashy cosmic oneness experience—one you'd probably think was the ultimate. But her awakening didn't last, because she hasn't been willing to feel lower vibrations, nor accept that she creates her life. "I didn't create my ex-husband . . ." "My dad is just an idiot. . ." I could only smile when she said about this book, "That book makes me feel things I don't like." She quit reading it. (We're still friends.)

Every teacher, medium, channel, psychic, indeed every human being, hears, sees, and feels different things when they talk to God, depending on their level of consciousness. The thing that is "true" at one level of consciousness is "less true" at a higher level of consciousness. It is very challenging to experience God fresh and uninfluenced by cultural images and myths, but I encourage you to aim for it. Your understanding of God evolves endlessly with Divine Openings.

I share with you some of my insights about Life, and it continues to evolve, as yours will. Your understanding of Life is filtered through your current level of consciousness, and will be only as high as your vibration is. What you "hear" God saying will always be colored by your vibration and your beliefs.

When someone says God said something angry, harsh or judgmental, that they got bad news from God, or that they experienced some negative manifestation of Spirit, that is just the highest voice of God they can hear at this time, at that level of consciousness. You cannot watch channel 24 television while your dial is tuned to the channel 7 frequency. You are getting the highest level you can from where you are at all times. Soften. Be open to a still-higher knowing, and be willing to let go of what you "knew." *Last year's guidance is already out of date.*

The authors of the ancient texts wrote at their current level of consciousness, and each translator after them colored their interpretation with their own consciousness, often with strong political agendas. It's easier to control people who don't know their true magnificence.

A teacher or medium with unresolved anger vibrations will hear an angry God and pass that message to her students. A teacher who has unresolved fear vibrations will channel messages of danger, violence, entities, evil spirits, and apocalypse, and urge you to take protective measures. A person with active sadness vibrations will give less positive messages about love and relationships. In my twenty-one days of silence in India, my past conditioning, emotional baggage, and spiritual concepts had to be emptied out before I could fully experience The All That Is without preconceptions. Will you let go of all the stuff in your mind now?

You have to at least be in the vibrational neighborhood of this material to even be able to hear it. It is more difficult to hear someone whose vibration is very much higher. Often a person who didn't get it before picks this book up again and says, "Why didn't I get this before?"

You will gradually upgrade your teachers, or begin to feel more like their peer, but you might want to stay in their orbit for fun. When your current teacher is no longer bringing you value, joy, laughter, or when their help doesn't fit or work for you anymore, you are complete with them. It is time to honor and appreciate them, and move on. Many of my past teachers are still beloved eternal companions in my heart, though I do not look to them for teaching now.

As I look back on my own evolution, I see how my view of things evolved with my consciousness. For example: relationships. I wrote a book called *Dating To Change Your Life*. It was a breakthrough for me and it helped many people. Now I look back on it and see that so many of the ideas, rules, and beliefs I developed back then no longer apply to me today. But for people at that level of evolution with relationships, the book is still a hugely valuable, life-changing experience! Life attracts the right people to each book.

One universal quality of a high-level teacher is simplicity. If the method or the message is very simple, direct, and effective, it is usually of a higher vibration. If it is complicated, technical, difficult, and you need the teacher's everlasting guidance, it is farther from the direct power of The Divine. The Divine needs no complicated processes, theories, or methodologies; its workings are elegantly efficient and fast (if you can let it be.)

Personally, I respect most those teachers whose message has a very high and positive vibration; I avoid doomsayers and purveyors of bad news. I continue to take occasional inspiration from those who are ahead of me, and listen to any messengers The Divine sends. A passing stranger, friend or street person sometimes delivers a surprise message from The Divine. These synchronicities are appreciated even more as we recognize that in the oneness, the "others" who are bringing the messages are also aspects of ourselves. Increasingly, I directly experience myself as an aspect of The Divine and so I most often go within for guidance or inspiration.

As I found in my twenty-one days of silence, the questions we ask before awakening, rather than getting answered, often just disappear or no longer matter. Accordingly, when we have direct experiences of God, we don't ask questions about God; we are too busy experiencing it. Divine Openings gives you direct experience. Just live it and it all unfolds. You can stop working at it.

You will soon have your own direct knowing, and you will go inside for most of your answers.

Designing Your Own Personal Relationship With God

BECAUSE THE VAST All That Is, the ultimate form of God, is so large, unknowable, and impersonal that we cannot possibly relate to it, our best way of "knowing" God is through the more personal forms that we can talk to. Going inside for your answers becomes easier when you can relate intimately to The Indweller, and when you can translate its pure vibrations to words you can understand. Man has sought relatable concepts of God since the dawn of consciousness, from the first Stone Age drawings, the rain and fertility gods, the many specialized Hindu deities, the Greek mythologies, the White Buffalo Woman of the Native Americans, to Jesus, and so on.

This more personal God does know us, and does care about us, and wants not only our survival, but also our joy and thriving. This more personal God created us, and each of us is a holographic locus of it. That is why each of us feels like the center of the Universe, and indeed we are. In reality there is only one "Being" in many unique and wondrous bodies and forms, each with the illusion of being separate.

The Indweller is willing to make itself known to us in a form we can embrace or relate to. To a Christian, it may make itself known as Jesus, the Holy Spirit, or The Lord. To an Indian, it might come as a specialized aspect like Krishna, Lord Ganesha, Lakshmi or Shiva. To a Buddhist, Buddha; to a New Age person, a white light; to a more scientific type, a formless Universal Intelligence. For a musician it might be felt in inspired music. You may know it as the life force, intuition, or consciousness. Others call it Nature. God doesn't quibble over the name we call; only man makes those kinds of ridiculous dogmatic judgments. God knows to whom we're talking.

In India, a most remarkable thing happened to my concept of God. I learned that God has no self-nature, but is what you believe God to be, and that the amount of Grace you are able to let in depends on the relationship you have. I had seen evidence of this before in my devout grandparents on my father's side, who indeed did always get what they asked their God to provide, even down to physical healings and miracles. However primitive their evangelical Hell and brimstone beliefs seemed to me, they had a personal relationship with their God that worked. As a child and a teen, I couldn't separate the good from the bad of it, and I couldn't relate to this judgmental God that my Assembly of God preacher grandfather talked about. Unfortunately, I threw out a God that could have supported me well in other ways.

It was thrilling and inspiring to learn two new names for God in India. While I never cared about Hindu traditions, these names forever changed my relating with The Divine, and helped me design a concept of God that I could actually walk and talk with like a friend:

Yathokthakari: One who does as is bidden.

Bhakti Paradina: One who is at the beck and call of the devotee.

What a concept—that God behaves according to our expectations and is actually willing to do what *we* want rather than dictating its will to us! It shouldn't be so surprising—reality bends itself to our beliefs. We rob ourselves of infinite possibilities by holding onto limiting concepts of God.

While I thought I had already ditched those negative concepts of God learned from childhood, and embraced a more progressive and inclusive God, I realized that the vast formless God I'd been trying to relate to was just too nebulous and impersonal, too large for me to really connect with in any personal way. No wonder the relationship had been cool and distant. Life is hot and close-up, and your God better be intense and real if it's going to compete with daily in-your-face-physical reality. My God had been less real than the very distracting outer reality, so my God had been weak, hard to connect with, ineffectual. I needed a God that was more up-close and personal. One of our challenges in the physical plane is to not let the material world become our God. Whatever has most of your attention, and whatever you give your power to—that's your God. When life circumstances are in your face, they can grab your focus and drown out your all-important internal God focus.

When we were children, it was very easy for our image of our parents to get transferred onto our image of God; not surprising—our parents *were* God to us—the conduit through whom all things seemed to flow for so many of our impressionable years. My father was an uncommunicative strong, silent type, so of course, my concept of God was like that. If your parents were non-judgmental and kind, encouraging and supportive, loving and wise, your concept of God is more likely to be very, very good. But if your parents were the average parents, you may need to toss out those less than positive unconscious perceptions of God and replace them with qualities you want in your God. Why? Because God behaves the way you expect, and life will bring you the consequences and the proof of your belief.

Since all this gets conditioned in us before we learn to use words, it can be invisible, hard to identify, so deeply ingrained that we don't even notice it. How could fish notice they are in water? No other reality is imaginable! You don't feel your clothes on your skin—you don't notice it because you've felt it all your life. We literally can't feel those early assumptions because we've never felt anything else and so have no contrast to compare them to. Most people never got the opportunity to clear that up—until now. It's not work, though. All you have to do is ask for Divine help, design your new concept of God, and God will do the rest. The Divine will even come to you if you are afraid of it, angry at it, or have doubts. Just ask.

I created a persona of God that I could really talk to and relate to; in effect, I designed my own ideal relationship with God, giving Him/Her all the qualities my heart desired, all the qualities my earthly parents didn't have, all that I had wanted from Life but hadn't received.

This was fun! I asked that "my" God relate to me with humor, playfulness, friendliness, and caring, in addition to all the expected qualities like unconditional love, all-knowingness, and power (but without being a bossy authority.) Later on I amended that to a God who cared about my every need, my every concern, who wanted to play with me and participate in every aspect of my life, who gives me messages I can understand, who loves to co-create with me, and who considers me a partner. God finally evolved into an inner friend who really listened and communicated back to me in signs, events, or in my own voice. This was quite different from the old one-way pleas to the angry, petty, judgmental God my grandfather had preached about. Grandpa meant well, but had told me that God condemned girls wearing pants, and while I had not exactly bought it, it had distanced me from that judgmental "God." I didn't even like the word God back then. Many still don't. Notice if you wince when you hear it. This new God needed me, valued me, and delighted in all my adventures, and even my mundane daily tasks. This continued to evolve for me until now I cannot even conceive of myself as separate from God, so it's hard to even call it a "relationship." Start where you are, talk to God constantly, and let it evolve.

Many people still have resistance to authority figures, and if you do, guess what? God seems like the ultimate authority figure, which puts big distance between you and God without your knowing it's happening. Take God out of the authority figure role and put God into the nurturing role if you want a more open, loving relationship.

With help from Divine Openings, God becomes a tangible reality, an experience instead of a concept, after this redesigning process. A humorous miracle during my silence brought it all home to me. I had a tiny flashlight I hung around my neck after "lights out" in the dark dorm room. Its little metal handle broke one day, and one piece of the metal was lost. I sat the flashlight on the dorm room nightstand overnight. The next morning the metal handle on the flashlight was fixed. It was whole; the missing piece had reappeared. There was no crack where the break in the handle had been. I laughed. My playful God had sent me a playful sign, and I understood. It said to me, "Everything is so assured for you now—there's nothing left for me to do for you but fix your flashlight." It also said, "Even this small detail of your life is so important to me that I will perform a miracle for you just to fix your flashlight." That tiny flashlight sits on my coffee table to this day, as a reminder. It brings tears of joy to remember.

If a voice inside feels good, I know it's my Large Self. If it feels bad, it's my small self. Minute by minute, day by day, my relationship with the Divine went vastly deeper than it had ever gone before.

The Divine will be whatever you want.

ACTIVITY: Write your latest concept of God in your notebook, and spend time talking to this new type of God, as you would build any new relationship. Continually create a new concept of God that works best where you currently are. It will change.

Your Desires Granted

TALK TO THE INDWELLER within you constantly. Any kind of communication will work. It's happy to hear from you. It doesn't quibble about how you address it, or whether you call it prayer or meditation or conversation, whether you word it properly, or write it down or not. Don't get hung up on words, processes, or rituals. Talk to God like a friend. Be yourself. You can even argue with God or get mad at God. Who could handle it better, or less judgmentally?

God is just happy to hear from you at all.

The Indweller knows your unspoken needs. When you feel bad, The Indweller hears that you want to feel good, and creates what you want. All you have to do it step into it. When you don't have what you want, The Indweller feels your wanting. I've had clients spontaneously heal from long-standing injuries during Divine Openings when they had not even told me the problem existed and they had not asked for healing. Divine Openings literally opens you up so the Grace that's always flowing to you can get in. Many complicated technologies have been devised—not understanding how simple it is to ask and receive. Once Divine Openings has opened that door for you, you just feel what you need and want, and let go, knowing it's coming.

The basic formula is: you ask (or feel a need), The Indweller answers, you let it in. Getting out of the way and learning to let go of resistance is your only job, but it takes practice. The Indweller always hears you ask, even if you don't say it in words, even if it's just a discomfort you feel or a desire deep inside, so the asking is automatic on your part. The Indweller always grants the essence of your request, and just waits for the crack of an opening to fulfill it in the material world. Grace does ninety percent. Your only job, your ten percent, is to get out of the way and let it in.

Grace does ninety percent. Your ten percent is to let it in.

Divine Openings fortunately helps you with the part humans have the most difficulty with: *getting out of the way*, and *letting it in*. When our pipes are shrunken, Grace can't get in as fully as it's offered. We ask and then don't let it in; we tense up and doubt, feel unworthy, focus on the lack of it, and so block its coming. Try this: tense up and clench your muscles, your jaw, ball up your fists. Imagine someone trying to give you something to make you feel better when you're like that. That's what resistance is. Now relax and hold out your open hands. Now you can receive. It's humanity's Ancient Mind conditioning that keeps us tense and resistant. We can't fix it ourselves, but Grace can, without effort. Just say yes. Say it out loud right now. *YES!* Keep saying yes.

I used to puzzle over why the Bible said that Jesus was the only way we could be "saved," since that seemed to exclude much of humanity who never heard about Jesus. I just could not see this Creator I know so intimately and personally leaving anyone out. Now I feel it meant that man has trouble doing it for himself because he's so stuck in the small separate self, that the Grace of the

Divine is the only thing powerful enough to do the job—that the only way out of suffering for humanity is awakening with the help of that Grace. Mere action on the mundane level won't do it. You are "saved" (helped) by Grace, by any name. You will soon experience what that means, regardless of your religion or path. You may even choose to become "the hands" that help bring it down to Earth. People the world over come to be initiated as Givers of Divine Openings.

Many of us now have the sort of relationship with The Presence that allows us to simply think of something, without formal prayer or process, and it comes. You can have that type of relationship too. This book will show you how, step by step. Let go of any concepts of a God who doesn't give you all you want. Those beliefs block your receiving. When your God is loving, kind, and supportive, everything you ask for is given. Because it fits your new belief, you can let it in.

When your God is that friendly to you, that intimately involved in your daily life, the essence of everything you ask for, no matter how mundane, is delivered. People who have this type of relationship with God don't have to pray, or write it down, or set goals; they simply ask casually, and Life Force fulfills the request, just as a doting earthly father, mother, or benefactor would. You can have such a relationship when you begin to regularly talk to God like your friend and confidant, and stop thinking of God as some authority figure, separate from you, uninterested in your mundane desires. Now I'm at a place where I rarely ask for anything; I let go and let God guide me in the best directions. But yesterday I did ask for rain, and then let go. With no rain in the forecast, it came by this morning, and the week's forecast is full of rain.

Let go of and replace any concept that you have to earn things, because if you have that concept, you will have to earn everything. Decide that God wants to grace you with everything you want, with ease. Remember, worthiness is not an issue to God. Unworthiness is a mind-construct. You are worthy just as the birds and flowers are worthy of their sustenance.

Let go of and replace any concept that you have been judged as unworthy, because if you believe that, it shrinks your pipes, and Grace can't get in as easily. Decide to agree with God that your worth is already a given. The very fact that you were given the gift of life proves your worthiness. Simply reading this book and receiving the Divine Openings in it will help you open up to know your worthiness and let in the Grace that is offered to you in every moment.

Let go of the belief that life is about lessons, because if you believe that, you will have lots of lessons, whereas if you believed life was about joy you'd have lots more joy. Life will evolve you, you'll learn and grow naturally, but this doesn't have to be some serious, dreary school! Decide that God wants you having fun as you evolve. You are actually closest to God when you're happy, and you'll soon know why.

Let go of and replace any concept that your worldly needs and desires are not important to God. If you think your daily needs are trivial to God, you can't let as much Grace in. The Presence, of which you are an integral part, does want you to have what you want in the material world, so the more you can get out of the way and let that in, the easier it can be delivered. People who have their material and relationship needs met are freer to fulfill their spiritual and service lives. One who is constantly struggling to make ends meet makes neither a good model for others, nor has much time or money to have a spiritual life and uplift others.

Create a new relationship with a God who's up close and personal.

If prayer feels intimate to you, pray, and know the answer is being given even if you know not yet what it is. The answer may not be a voice or a vision; it is more often a feeling, a knowing, a simple thought—or later, an event or person just shows up. Listen, watch, feel and appreciate it now—in advance, which speeds the arrival of it.

Taking It Inside To The Presence

THE MAIN PURPOSE of my long period of silence in India was to spend all my time communing with The Indweller; to take it all inside to The Divine Presence—the feelings, the thoughts, the questions—to talk with The Presence within like a dear friend. I got answers (usually non-verbal), was nurtured, and developed that intimate relationship at a deeper, more tangible level than ever before. By avoiding even eye contact, I kept my focus inward. How often do we give our whole being and our undivided attention to The Presence for even one day?

To me it was delicious to be silent—the ultimate vacation! The growing relationship with my beloved Divine Presence within became too precious to even consider breaking the silence. It was like the intense first few weeks of a romantic relationship where your attention and focus is given only to the beloved, except this time it was the ultimate Beloved within. The deeper into that silent embrace I dived, the sweeter it felt, and the stronger I became. It was ultimate fulfillment.

Once that relationship with The Indweller was established, the rest came easy. I noticed that those of us who took all our feelings, challenges and questions inside to The Divine had profound experiences, while those who turned outside to other people never developed that depth of communion with The Indweller nor tapped their internal power.

Some of the participants could not bear the silence, and by venting their feelings and thoughts to other people they perpetuated the old strategies they had used all along to avoid deep feeling and keep their story running. I was tired of my stories and I didn't want to tell them ever again. Long before India I had been teaching that telling our negative stories strengthens the unwanted reality. The stories give the negative reality more juice and drain our power. When I dropped the stories and took any negative feelings into that intimate communion within, by Grace, The Divine did all the heavy lifting. Things I had struggled with for years evaporated like mist.

Notice how trivial and ineffectual most talk is, how it leaks our energy, takes us out of the moment. Notice how we use talking to run from feelings, even as we're talking about feelings! Talking about feelings was replaced with silently feeling them all the way through. I lost my taste for counseling as I experienced an increasingly strong desire to take everything to The Presence Within. When you're truly free, counseling and getting "healed" makes absolutely no sense. I marveled at the lightning speed with which my requests were being fulfilled. Now I notice that my clients and audiences experience the same thing.

There had long been a desire to stop looking to any outer source for answers, comfort, information and direction. It was a dream come true. Once I was out of the way, The Grace that's always been raining could get in. Everything I asked for came, some things in an instant, others in good time. I became so confident that all things were coming that my old habit of doubting just *disappeared*. It never even occurred to me to work on myself ever again once I realized I was on an evolutionary fast track that required me to do nothing but pay attention and stay awake.

This habit of going within for all needs has persisted long since the twenty-one days of silence. The Divine is right here and will answer any need quickly, accurately and fully, from its unlimited resources and all-encompassing knowledge. All I have to do is relax and get out of the way. I might still ask for practical advice or help on matters of worldly expertise. The Divine might send any type of answer through another person. God knows I still call tech support, although even for that, I might first close my eyes, still my mind, and receive inspiration; or get my vibration in receiving mode so I'll let the help or answer in. I often get inner answers, or the problem resolves itself!

There is something you can always rely on, and it is found inside of you.

A Relationship With The Divine In Good Times

IN A CARTOON by Tex Reid, a cowboy walks into church and tips his hat to the preacher, who says, "What is it this time, Clem? Drought? Drop in cattle prices? Land taxes got raised?" After seeing how nurturing, how fun, how practical my new relationship with God was, I decided never again to relegate my communication with it to those times when I needed help. I knew God wouldn't judge me if I did that, but it was me who'd miss out. Now there is an ongoing, minute-by-minute dialogue, even when I'm communing with people, animals, and nature, or working with my computer or driving my car. God is everywhere and everything. Life is that communion. Meditation is great for the pure joy of it, or to simply rest in the deep silence of the Void. It is more refreshing than sleep. Do it to reset, refresh or get empty, not to fix things or get somewhere.

People talk about meditating to save the planet. Get happy, radiate happiness, and that contributes high vibrations to the planet more than you know. Meditating from "there's something wrong with the planet," just creates more of that, and more discord in you. It can actually make it worse.

Although I'm usually naturally in the flow, some days I pre-pave my day, letting go so The Divine can line it all up for me, and so I can recognize all opportunities to make the day fulfilling and joyful, efficient and constructive. Once I've asked for something I never ask again, because if it's not here the only thing in the way is my own resistance—so I ask only for release of resistance regarding things I've asked for that haven't arrived. This creative, proactive focus has replaced the old fixing mindset, and problem solving is not the focus of my life. Sometimes I wake so clear about what to do that I just leap up and launch into it.

We are moving toward a new world that is based on *creation rather than fixing or problem solving.* Feel the difference. This is key.

Fixing, preventing, and surviving are of the old paradigm. We cannot see the solution while we're still in the same consciousness that created it. Our dialogues with God soon transcend asking for help (as child asks parent) and become more of a co-creative process (as with an equal.) The small self will tell you that you still need to keep seeking, defending, and solving problems. The mind is a wrong-seeking missile! It knows that once you are a free, empowered, creative being, the small self will no longer be in control.

Freedom from seeking and fixing is a strange and impossible concept for many, and it may seem incomprehensible at first. After a lifetime of struggle, overcoming, fixing, and earning, it may seem odd to simply hop on a new wave and be carried to wherever and whatever you want. What will life be about when you're not seeking enlightenment, striving to fulfill desires, trying to fix problems, or get somewhere—when all your basic needs are met? It's exciting to wonder, and out of that wondering will come your next steps.

If you could create anything you wanted, not out of need, but just for the joy of it (and you can and you will), what would it be? The Level 2 Online Course goes deeply into creation and fun, after you're mostly out of suffering and ready to play on this Earth!

Commune in good times too! There are going to be a lot of them!

The Questions Cease

DURING THE TWENTY-ONE DAYS of silence, we were occasionally given a half-hour to talk with our guides, who were essentially monks. We all had questions to ask of them, and some participants were like kids in a candy store stuffing themselves with all the goodies they could. But I was clear that I came there to find answers within, and I was soon guided from within to stop asking them, and to begin to take my questions directly to The Divine. Suddenly answers appeared to questions I had pondered for decades. "Why had I become fearful years before when I saw a brilliant white beam of light in meditation, and again while out camping?" The answer came from within: the small self interprets everything unknown through a filter of fear. I remembered Bible stories I'd read as a child where people nearly always fell down in fear and covered their eyes when confronted with an angel. Our small self is afraid of our own light, and anything unfamiliar!

On about the ninth day, even my incessant internal questions to The Divine about life, love, money, the future, and the meaning of it all suddenly ceased—for the first time in my life. There was an eerie silence in my head. Rather than getting "answered," most of the questions simply lost their meaning or evaporated as my mind became empty and still. I reported to the guides I had no more questions and didn't need to meet with them anymore. I realized that most of our questions are just the mind doing its thing. The mind questions and doubts—that's just what it does. When the mind stops its chatter, and we are still, we can simply *be*.

All was quiet inside me, and I would sit and marvel at the unaccustomed space inside my head. Any newly arising question was either answered immediately and definitively by the Divine within, or was quickly recognized as meaningless intellectual jabber. It became humorously clear that Life doesn't have a why. *Life is.* Life is for living, or as my friend Penny used to say, "Life just lifes." Asking questions, analyzing, trying to figure it out, naming it, and categorizing it are mind-distractions from actual living. People who are truly living don't ponder the meaning of life—they're living! They experience each moment. "Why?" Ask a bird why it lives.

I would never have such big questions again. My questions are now practical. "What do I do today?" "What would feel good?" "What will I create next?" "What's an easier way to get this done?" Now the answers just come or I drop the question and let go.

I became so empty that hours and days would pass with scarcely a thought rippling the surface of my mind. It was bliss. When I returned home to regular life, while my mind would occasionally get cluttered, it cleared out again as I took it to The Divine, laid it down, and found stillness again. Soon a rhythm was established, thoughts came and went, leaving a clean slate for the next moment.

There were still moments of confusion, but I knew that meant I needed to sit quietly, slow down, and let the space clear again. Then I could discern the answer, or once again the question would simply lose meaning as a new consciousness opened up. Problems exist only in the consciousness that created them. In the brighter light of a new consciousness, the old questions don't even make sense—they're non-issues. For example, when governments try to agree on what to do about nuclear weapons within the defensive and survival-based consciousness that created those weapons, all you get is laws and regulations that partially work or don't work, and no one feels safe to follow them. In an expanded consciousness, people wouldn't even think of using those weapons. Questions of who should have what kind, and how to regulate them, seem pretty pointless from that new consciousness. They look back and wonder why it wasn't obvious sooner.

In most countries, a heightened consciousness about women has resulted in better treatment, equality and voting rights. The previous consciousness didn't support those possibilities. Suddenly, it seems very natural. Leaps in consciousness are birthed in a few people at first, in a few countries, then it spreads to others, then finally, the entire material world changes to match. You are a frontrunner for changes in consciousness. If it feels like it's taking too long, remember that evolution will go on forever. In the universal sense, there is no rush and no finish.

Once home, the help was always here for me even if it was just a soothing feeling. Sometimes the answer was clear information, sometimes it was a feeling of, "just wait, be happy, it will be alright," sometimes it was an action to take right now. The result was profound in my new work; guidance poured in. You do need to take action when guided. This is a material world!

People asked me, "How do you know which thoughts are from The Divine and which ones are just noise?" I had not been able to answer that until I knew it from direct experience. Every one of us is constantly receiving communication, inspirations, nudges, whispers and suggestions from the Divine, but when our minds are cluttered and our eyes are focused on problems and distractions, those inspired thoughts land in a din of loud thought-chatter, and sorting through that to find which thoughts are the inspired ones is difficult, especially since the Divine often whispers soothingly instead of shouting. Guidance isn't often delivered by a burning bush and a booming voice. But it became easy to recognize the subtle, quiet, Divinely inspired thoughts from within my new quiet, clear mind. They always feel good, and are always good news.

In the stillness you can hear the voice of God.
It may sound just like you, except smarter.

A Second Chance For A Happy Childhood

ON ABOUT THE FIFTEENTH DAY of the twenty-one days I literally became a little girl again. I put my hair in pigtails, walked like a little girl, looked like a little girl, and felt as innocent as any fresh-faced child. When a woman walking by broke the eye contact taboo to laugh at my pigtails, I stuck my tongue out at her, and she giggled! I laughed at myself, realizing it was the authentic response of a five year old. I laughed again when Marian, who was seventy-four years old, stuck her tongue out at me a week later! We were all returning to innocence.

Splashing through puddles on the large lawn in front of the women's dormitory, laughing at frogs poking their heads out from the crevices, singing songs to myself, talking softly out loud to The Presence, it was a softer, gentler childhood than the first one. There was unconditional love and support, and this time the voices from within were soothing and wise, and unlike my first childhood, there were no voices outside me to drown them out. Love had a chance.

There's an innocent child within you still.

Fear Of The Unknown

YOU MAY HAVE a number of steps to take before you are ready to let go of old vibrational habits, past hurts, working on yourself, and other baggage. Be easy about it. The less you push, the easier and faster it goes. Don't resist your resistance.

At one point it seemed the one thing still holding me back was my small self's fear of letting go of that last chunk of control. We know that our letting go to the larger flow of Life, or God—whatever you prefer to call it—is a key to freedom. The Divine beckons us to turn our plane and go with the tailwind, but won't force us to, or take our Free Will away. The small self values its struggle and does not want to give it up because that's the end of its game.

We get to choose how much to let go, and when to put the small self in the back seat and let The Divine take the wheel. The small self may or may not throw little fits at times, just when you thought you had let go. But don't add more resistance to resistance! Be easy on yourself, have fun.

The day after the twenty-one day process was over, we were all at the beach, resting, knowing that the enlightenment process had begun but was far from over. I shared with Marian that I was still somewhat afraid of losing my small-self identity. She gave a snort, smirked, and said, "After seventy four years of it, I'm sick of it. I'll be happy to see it go!"

It was a pivotal moment for me; I could feel how in all her seventy four years, her small self being in control had never gotten her all of what she wanted. She was ready to let go to the flow of life. I didn't know which I was more afraid of, having my small self take a back seat, or having it keep driving! The small self actually gets very happy once you let go. It wasn't so bad after all.

The liberation I received there I will be eternally grateful for. Other elements of it I was soon guided to leave behind. Making the guru into God didn't work for me. God is within each of us equally. No matter how powerful a teacher is, never give your power to them. I see my job as guiding you to remember who you are, and helping you claim your own power. I graciously declined every offer to give power to the gurus, each time choosing to turn to The Divine within.

People have asked me why I came home with more power than others who were initiated there. Slowly *feel* each one of my answers: 1) I gave no power away to anyone and focused solely inward in the silence. 2) I let go of everything I knew, and got empty. "You must come as a little child to enter the Kingdom of Heaven." 3) I didn't try to figure it out, but went into no-mind, a very powerful state of direct knowing, beyond rational thinking. 4) I stopped seeking.

No More Working On Yourself

BEFORE I GIVE you any methods, I want to make sure you've completely let go of working on yourself—so you don't cram Divine Openings into the tired old "work on yourself" paradigm. The old paradigm of lifetimes of working on yourself, learning "lessons," clearing karma, or healing yourself are the polar opposite of Divine Openings. This is all for joy, and it leads to more joy. I know I've said this, but sometimes it takes a while for readers to let it in. It really is possible to enjoy the Divine Openings processes, relax into them, they work, and *that's it*.

Let go and let The Divine do the heavy lifting, and whatever you're struggling with lifts or shifts. Divine Openings is pleasure, not work. If you work on yourself, or give your power to someone else to work on you, it actually reverses your progress.

Here's the "cowgirl guru" speaking: Get a life—outside of spiritual seeking that is. If your social life revolves around sessions, talking about issues, giving and receiving emotional support, discussing new modalities, going to metaphysical meetings, meditations, seminars, and working on yourself, *get a real life!* Share about this book, and soon friends and family won't want to talk about problems, issues, what's wrong, or lack either. Do real hobbies, and have fun. Get a life outside of work, too. Lighten up and live. We all got on a spiritual path to get happy and have a great life, right? You can begin to live now.

Someone asked, isn't all Divine Energy the same? No. There are different frequencies, just as radio stations broadcast different frequencies. Some are far more powerful than others, and do different things. Would you listen to two radios at once, even if both stations are good? Spiritual/metaphysical people who do too many energies, books, and modalities have a discordant vibration, but don't know it. If you feel resistance to letting it be as simple and easy as Divine Openings is, just keep reading, and letting Grace in. It gets clear as you awaken fully.

Notice your dreams, which may change dramatically with Divine Openings. Any "bad dreams" are releasing resistance for you. We used to think we had to interpret or work at dreams, but Divine Openings has taken the work out of that too. There's nothing to an alyze or do. You get benefits whether you remember the dream or not. Much of the "work" in this process is done in your dreams or in sleep when you're least resistant. Let it be that easy.

You may be kept awake in strange states. Just lie there, relax, breathe, snuggle yourself, and savor. Don't resist being awake and you'll get up rested. "Insomnia" is just another brand of resistance. We have Divine Openings Givers who now only sleep a couple of hours a night—they glow and have boundless energy. It isn't insomnia. I've laid awake all night receiving a download for a seminar and felt wonderful all day the next day. Relax. Let it be.

Divine Opening

SIT QUIETLY and contemplate the image for two minutes.
Don't work or try. Just open to Divine Grace. Then close your eyes and lie down
for at least fifteen to twenty minutes—longer if you can.

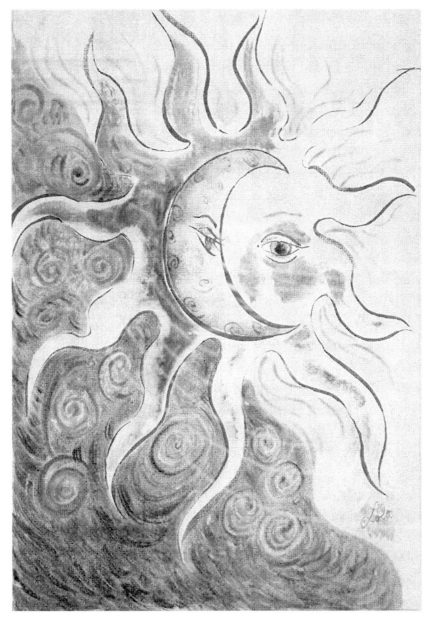

Figure 3—Solstice, an ink drawing by Lola Jones.

Lay It All Down At The Feet Of The Divine

HAVING NEVER CARED for rituals, at first I merely tolerated the ancient Hindu rituals we did in India. Some were simple, and some were hours long and incomprehensibly complex. While I recognized their value, could feel their beauty and power, appreciated the thousands of years and the generations of masters that had left their legacy in these rituals, and especially appreciated the time and passionate energy the monks spent in doing fire ceremonies for us in the oppressive heat, I planned on leaving all that in India and having a more simple and direct relationship with God, sans rituals, back at home. On some level, doing anything that is too complicated feels like giving my power away to it. In my heart I knew my relationship with my Inner Source need never be hard or complicated. It is simple and it is right here in any moment—no special rituals or props required.

One ritual did touch me profoundly and stayed with me. Each morning as we began our day, one of the monks sang a chant in some soaring, otherworldly voice; and the arati was performed (a devotional waving of the lighted oil lamp before the altar.) It was not the arati that touched me so deeply; it was the prostration at the end of the arati. When prostrating, we laid our bodies face down, stretched out full length on the straw mats, foreheads flat on the floor, with palms together pointing toward the altar. (This ritual will be explained for you in greater detail later.)

I was unwilling to prostrate to an altar to the guru, as was suggested—I don't use an altar nor give any power to props or objects. Instead, I turned my devotion directly to The Divine Within. The prostration became for me symbolic of letting go to the flow of life, of my merging back into Source, and a way to release resistance. During the twenty-one days when we prostrated (maybe thirty times total) each time my forehead touched the floor I heard my body sigh more and more deeply. Sometimes I felt some old burden or unnamable heaviness being laid down as I whispered through tears of relief, "Thank you that it isn't my job to figure *this* out anymore." Or "Thank God I don't have to carry *that* heavy weight anymore, whatever it was."

You may lay all the heaviness down now.

My forehead coming to rest on the floor became a cue for my entire body to relax to a degree I had never before experienced. Tensions, burdens, fears, and limitations I had been carrying for God knows how long melted away—no work, no understanding, no processing. Eventually I must have laid it all down; my body relaxed to an astounding extent. This release of resistance showed up in many ways, but one tangible way was that my hips became so flexible and free, and swayed so much when I walked that I felt boneless. My hip never popped again. It was a delight just to feel my body glide along the long gravel road from the dorm to the meditation hall. A body worker asked me after the program how I got so loose; she had never seen anyone walk with such freedom in their hip joints, even after extensive body work. She wanted to know my secret. I told her, "It's release of resistance! It's letting go." Many there unfortunately didn't know about resistance.

Afterwards, at the beach at Mahabalipuram, it was again demonstrated to me just how relaxed and alive my body was. Someone well recommended offered me a massage for ten dollars American.

I looked at him blankly, as if the very idea of needing relaxation did not compute. My head fell back as I smiled a big toothy smile. I could not comprehend wanting a massage. I went for a blissful walk on the beach instead, still smiling at the thought and marveling at the pleasure I felt in my body. After the thirty-two hours of travel home, I was not tired, stiff or jet lagged. My body is still in that relaxed state most of the time now. If it's not, I deliberately let go.

Dr. Hans Selye is commonly known as the father of modern stress management, and in the 1950s he demonstrated that the brain of the average normal person operates in a chronic state of survival stress that would be perfectly appropriate in a life-threatening situation, like fighting a lion or running from a bear. Worse, we have become so accustomed to it that we think it is normal. Everyone accepts it. It was only after releasing that tension that I finally knew what a relaxed body could feel like, and that was my new "normal" point. To this day I maintain a much, much lower baseline of stress. I can sit at the computer and get tense shoulders and simply release that tension by intention. If I want help I get bodywork. And since we can pass along evolutionary advances to others, my audiences pick this up very quickly. Many completely "lose" their capacity to maintain a steady state of stress in one or two sessions. I look forward to hearing how this goes for you.

The relaxing of tension was the first of many increasingly pleasurable realizations of just how physical the phenomenon of enlightenment is. The more it unfolds, the more I experience it as a full body phenomenon. It's not transcending the body, ascending out of the body, or conquering the body; it is fully inhabiting the body, fully experiencing the body, beyond any sensory experience I've ever had. It's having almost orgasmic ecstasy in mundane moments, finding profound pleasure in simple experiences, or streaming tears of profound bliss for no reason. It's a lightening up of the physical while simultaneously being more grounded.

But When Will I Be Done On This Planet?

WHEN I WAS a child I thought for sure I had landed on the wrong planet. I know many people who have had this experience of feeling out of place, and many who still do. "Who *are* these people who claim to be my family?" It is true that the earth plane can feel dense and heavy compared to the non-physical realm where the greater part of us lives, but once we know how this physical space/time reality works, its joys are great—so great that the Larger non-physical aspect of us clamors to come here repeatedly.

People only ask the question, "When do I graduate from Earth life and never have to come back?" when they feel separated from God. When there is suffering, of course people wish for rest and deliverance. Once there is no suffering, there is no desire to leave here. Here is as good as anywhere. You got on the ride—now you get to enjoy it.

There is nothing to graduate from, as there was never a test to pass. You don't earn your way out of here. That's that belief in "life as school" I was so happy to drop. When we know who we are and we are one with Divine Presence, we thoroughly enjoy this life, and are eager to return. You can skip school and go straight to the playground you so eagerly anticipated when coming here. We came here positive and full of plans, open and one with everything.

People who talk about wanting to ascend out of the body or who wish to leave this physical dimension have obviously not experienced a fully awake body and a fully flowered heart! There is usually a lot of pain in that body and heart, so of course they want to leave it.

Along with many other spiritual myths (search "spiritual myths" on our site) we were told this body is somehow less spiritual than being non-physical. This time/space reality is on the leading edge of creation, it's "where it is at," and we are deeply blessed to be here at this time. There may be a time to move on to other dimensions of life, but when you do, it will be with the joyful farewell of a powerful and fulfilled being, not the retreat of a victim who suffered enough.

It is inconceivable to ever imagine "finishing" anything in an eternal universe. When you live in bliss and peace and love you won't be worrying about fixing something in yourself or others. And you won't want to be rescued from this life—you will be truly living and enjoying it.

Life continues to flow in a never-ending stream of creation. You will increasingly create joyful and wonderful things, and then let them go. You will no longer resist anything or try to hold onto anything—you won't push it away and neither will you cling to it. One of the hallmarks of enlightenment is not just acceptance of or enduring what is, but authentically experiencing the beauty and perfection of what is. Of course, you cannot create this with your mind, or pretend you feel it when you don't. Just relax, enjoy the ride, and allow it to happen. It will.

This time/space reality is the hottest game going, although it gets weary being here if we constantly fly into headwinds. Let go, let it take you, and it becomes a tailwind. After death we release all resistance. Then we line up bright and fresh to come back and give it another go, optimistic that next time we'll be able to remember, follow our inner knowing, and go with the current. From our non-physical perspective before we came into physical manifestation, we were eager to experience the wonders of physicality, and we excitedly anticipated its pleasures and contrasts, knowing fully the challenges and possibilities of the game. You can enjoy it now!

Part of the game is to pretend we don't know who we are, and to discover it again—to go to sleep and then wake up. Babies love the peek-a-boo game where they cover their eyes, then peek through their hands. We are created in the image and likeness of our Creator, who also loves hide and seek games, adventures, and challenges. Most of all, The Creator loves to create.

True, once we get here and encounter the density of this plane, it can be hard to maintain the high vibration we intended. We encounter discord, confused energy, other people who are not aligned with Pure Source, and it's easy to get distracted. To lose our fresh innocence, get bogged down and burdened by the thoughts and conditioning of society and other humans. It can seem like a bad idea to have come here.

As babies emerge from floating in the womb and feel the density of the material plane, their vibration drops a bit, and they cry. They're still quite open and One with Life Source. And then well-meaning people begin to teach them how to "protect themselves," what horrors to avoid, "how life works" and how tough it is. They lose their positive expectation bit by bit and begin to focus on things they do not want, and the downward spiral away from their Pure Essence begins. They lose their focus on their own inner knowing, start listening to other "more experienced" beings and stop trusting their own guidance. They stop moving toward what feels good.

As a result, many people, especially spiritual people, begin to feel that they are "in the wrong place" or "on the wrong planet" or that this place is "bad" and needs fixing. When we return to the place of innocence and trust and connection, we are happy on this planet, with all its contrasting experiences, knowing we can choose, and that our safety is ultimately guaranteed. The "worst" that can happen to us is that we return fully to our non-physical, unlimited, Large Self.

From that broader perspective, we relish Earth life, and are secure in the knowledge that even if we splat, we'll be back again for another ride, to take the experiment on to yet another level. We know we can do even more next time because all the desires that don't get fulfilled in this life carry over into the next. That's how evolution works. That's how the exponential growth of recent years happened. That's how kids recently born can use a computer by age three. Desires carry over from generation to generation and often get fulfilled by the next generation. The desires of past generations had built up to the point where a critical mass occurred. Even if they died before they ever got their desires, we're now reaping the benefits of that. The animal kingdom does this too.

After reawakening, you will not wish to be elsewhere. You'll be too busy living. The fully awake Divine Presence in you appreciates the opportunity to experience physical creation in the full sensory richness that only physical incarnation can provide!

You're in the right place! And it's about to get really fun!

The End of Drama

VEILS LIFT AND things are seen that were invisible before, and there's no going back unless you choose to. One unforgettable day long before Divine Openings came along, I remember having a flat empty feeling once there was no more drama in my life. I had ended an unhappy and dramatic relationship and begun a course of sane and proper dating with sane and suitable men. Looking back it was easy to see the old drama for what it was, and it was not pretty. The desperate "love," the fighting, conflict, complaining and commiserating, the longing and suffering and the extreme charge on those radical emotions now felt violent and unsavory to me. Drama feeds the small self a steady diet of raw fuel that perpetuates more drama. The endless conversations with friends to "solve problems" were no more than gasoline on the fire.

The evaporation of drama addiction left a void where before there had been zing and pop and zap. I didn't want it back, but I felt somehow lacking in what I had thought was passion. A teacher at the time told me that I could deliberately create a whole new kind of passion and excitement, comparable to developing a new taste for gourmet vegetable dishes when the taste buds were jacked up on cookies, ice cream, cake and greasy junk food. The vegetables taste pretty bland at first, but after a while, you can taste every nuance of them and savor every subtle flavor. The occasional taste of sugary junk food actually becomes unpleasant. When drama did occasionally make a brief appearance after that, it was quite distasteful, and I recoiled quickly, thanking God for the rich, wholesome sweetness of my new drama-free, no-suffering life.

The End Of Seeking At Last!

YET ANOTHER VEIL was lifted during my three-week silence, and behind it at first was also emptiness. So much of my life had been spent seeking—seeking God, seeking answers, seeking my dreams, that when that seeking was over, as happens to many people, I scarcely knew what to do. My friend Bob once said about his girlfriend, "If she wasn't a seeker, a recovering something-or-other, and a 'survivor' of something, she wouldn't know who she was." It had almost come to that for me too. I identified so much with the search that the end of it was inconceivable. As my small self slowly relaxed and let go over the ensuing months, I realized that seeking is a way for the small self to hold on, to stay in control. If the small self can perpetuate an incessant search, it can stay in the driver's seat and continue the charade of seeking relief, while it addictively creates more problems to struggle against, more paths to check out, more excuses not to arrive. Once the search is over, and the Large Self is driving, the small self has to take a back seat and let go. There is not much left for it to do, nothing more for it to pretend it's trying to solve.

There is an old story about a seeker who comes unexpectedly to a door in the woods that says, "God lives here. Welcome, come on in." Elated, the seeker walked up to the door and raised his hand to knock, and then thought twice. He sat on the step perplexed. Soon he stood up, turned around, and walked on down the path. He could not give up the addiction of seeking.

I was ready to give it up. I had thoroughly kicked the drama addiction, and was deliberately set on the end of seeking—ready for life to be about creating, expanding, playing, enjoying and loving.

Once I returned home from the twenty-one days of silence, for the first time in years, I began to wake in the mornings with my mind at peace. It felt a bit empty sometimes, at first. I was accustomed to a mind filled with problems needing to be solved. But there was no hurry to fill this empty space. I let it evolve naturally, and spent a few days in the emptiness, lying on the sofa, barely interested in eating or doing anything except feeling and breathing, which suddenly seemed like brand new discoveries.

And then one day my body started wanting to move about and my mind began to generate some newly productive thoughts. Eventually I knew what to do—I began living and creating instead of seeking! Each day I did what I was guided to do, doing my best at any given moment to get out of the way, and things started to happen, even where there had been stagnation before.

When talking about what I wanted, I had been for some time using the metaphor of how birds fly in a flock at high speeds, swooping and turning and whirling, yet wonder of wonders, they never bump into each other or crash. While scuba diving, I've watched fish in giant schools as big as a house swimming millimeters from each other, but never bumping into each other, turning in unison -- separate, but all moving as one.

My wish came true. Life began to flow in that easy way much more often. Now I know that there is a unified field that connects all life, and the invisible force that orchestrates everything guides all beings *that let go and flow with it*. With steadily increasing ease the inspired thoughts, the solutions, the people, and the circumstances would line up for me to produce the result needed for everyone involved. My only job was to let go and relax, feel good, and let the Universe line it all up for me. There was awareness that I still had a distance to go in my journey to enlightenment, yet I felt complete ease in putting one foot in front of the other without striving or stressing about it. I didn't "know" more or have any more "answers" than before; I couldn't see farther ahead than about two stepping-stones in front of me. Nevertheless, I walked with a buoyant feeling that everything was not only all right, but perfectly in order.

During that pre-menopausal crash and long dark slump a few years before, I had wondered if I would ever recover my enthusiasm and confidence. Divine Openings renewed me at age fifty-two—and soon had me on fire with inspiration. I could hardly wait to get into action each day. Things unfolded with amazing velocity. Creativity overflowed in new and delightful forms.

Within seven weeks after the twenty-one days, starting from zero, I had a busy life, full of networking, events, parties, speaking engagements and private clients. I gave Divine Openings every chance I got, and in three months I had given them to about three hundred people. I was more active and inspired than I had been in years, and sometimes worked tirelessly twelve to sixteen hours a day. It was guided action, inspired action. It felt good. Once things were launched and on a steady course, the work diminished and I had lots of playtime. To everything there is a season.

Now you can live and evolve instead of seeking.

Adjusting to the New Energies

UPON ARRIVAL HOME from India, I laid on the sofa vibrating for about three days, just being, and adjusting to the strange new sensations and perceptions. A friend who lived with me said, "Hey, I don't know what you're thinking or feeling, or what's going on." I looked at him with a glint of mischief in my eye and said, "Here, I'll share the contents of my mind with you." Then I gave him the blankest stare for about thirty seconds. After a few seconds, he got it and laughed—there was absolutely nothing going on in my mind to share, which explained why I had little interest in talking. *The fresh new pure experience of Life was so rich that talking about it paled.* I rarely talk about "it" now except while teaching. It feels better to experience it than to talk about it.

The funny thing is that no matter how astounding, how mind-blowing the elevated states are when we first achieve them, they soon come to feel quite normal to us. A man commented that I had touched his shoulder in passing behind him at a public event, and that he had felt an electric buzz that made him jump and turn around to see who it was. Divine Openings Givers often feel that electrical buzz when we get a new "energy download," but in that moment I was feeling quite normal. My vibration felt extraordinary to him by contrast (it's all relative) while it felt ordinary to me. Someone will comment how lit up I am, and I might be feeling rather tired in that moment. I am just used to being lit up and it feels like no big deal.

A client marveled at how, after one session, her endometriosis had cleared up, and for the first time in years, she is not balled up in pain during her menstrual cycle with her brain incapable of working. Instead, she is happy and energetic. She has felt more at ease than she has felt in years, and her mind is not making up stories of what might happen, like it used to do. Her eyes are bright and clear, where before she had looked dull and low energy.

When I seemed to take it all in stride, she leaned forward and beamed, "This is amazing. This is a miracle!" Then I started laughing. I said, "I know that incredible as all of this is to you, it happens so often now that I think it's just normal! I do appreciate it and thank The Divine every day, but it is no longer so surprising." I was glad she had made such a point of it; it gave me a new chance to see it afresh and rave about it.

By the time your enlightenment has unfolded considerably, you will accept it as normal, and you will quickly become accustomed to each of the higher states you achieve, and you will always want more. I remind my audiences of this, because they expect to keep feeling the awe and wonder daily, and that may not happen every day unless you make a point to focus on it and rave about it, because that level of awe and wonder will become normal for you. You feel it most each time you come to yet a higher state and it is new again. Raving brings it back.

This is apparently the ongoing reality for us as we evolve. Creation is never done. It wasn't done with the dinosaurs and it isn't going to be done with us. We will never be "done," even after we've achieved a huge degree of enlightenment. We won't be "seeking" in that old lackful way, but we will be expanding, creating, evolving, moving, elevating, just as the Universe continues to expand.

Seeking feels like there's a lack of something, or trying to fix something, get something or get somewhere. Expanding feels like the natural urge to keep joyfully evolving, just because it's our eternal nature. You celebrated high school graduation, and then you went to college. You celebrated your first great job, perhaps your marriage and the birth of children. And you're still not done expanding. Divine Openings keeps expanding you if you'll let go and fly with it.

Humans "habituate" to things, whether it is ecstasy or pain, and no matter how intense a sensation is, if it continues, it eventually feels normal. You've experienced this with a big new purchase that you've wanted for a long time. At first it seems so exciting to own that new computer with all the fancy features. You gaze at it in awe. "Wow, I can't believe I got this." Within a month or so it seems like no big deal. Sometimes I literally vibrate with newly downloaded frequencies—then I get used to it. As you unfold it is your natural state that you're returning to, after all.

The ecstatic peak states you may experience at times are not states our bodies are currently designed to sustain all of the time. While they've wonderful, it's best to enjoy them and let them ebb and flow. Don't get attached to anything. There can also be a small-self tendency to want the old familiar lows back. The small self is afraid of its own light!

At first, the regularly downloaded energy was intense at times. Sometimes it felt like pressure, like trying to squeeze more energy through the pipes than their diameter would allow, and at other times like an agitated buzzing, or an over-amping sensation. But as my capacity to hold that volume of flow and voltage increased, the pressure subsided. When I feel it increasing now, as it regularly does, I know more is trying to come through, and that my small self is resisting—I know to breathe for pleasure, take a hot bath, exercise, do something that feels good. Now I know how to let go and let it flow. We must let ourselves keep expanding. Resisting hurts, and it's supposed to!

The new energies may feel unfamiliar at first, then will become normal to you.

The Present Moment Takes Hold

IT BECAME INCREASINGLY hard to dwell on the past or the future as the present became rich and fully captivating. Friends and I would laugh so hard our stomachs cramped, and then the next day not be able to remember what we were laughing about, and it didn't seem to matter. We knew that equally funny, if not funnier things would occur tomorrow. And they did. There was no hanging on to anything. Losses were forgotten just as quickly. Yes, a few people may accuse you of not caring about anything or anyone. They won't understand until they're where you are that suffering over losses, setbacks or insults is simply a symptom of disconnection from your Large Self. There is truly no such thing as loss from The Large Self's standpoint, but even if you have some temporary sense of loss, your Large Self will find a way to fill in the gap if you allow it. One "downside"? When you live in the moment, if you're not aligned with your Large Self right now, it will feel really bad (and it's supposed to feel bad.) It may feel as if this moment will never end—as if this moment is all there is. Because this moment, the eternal now, *IS all there is.*

The Divine is always offering blessings in every moment, and as soon as we let go of the grip on the past, we have an open hand to extend to accept that new gift. Singer/songwriter, turned author, turned 2006 Texas gubernatorial candidate Kinky Friedman says it the down home Texas way:

When the horse dies, get off.

The Amazing Power Of Humor

KINKY'S QUOTE IS a good segue way into the next topic: humor. Humor has been a most cherished element of my life for some years now. I already shared with you about creating my own concept of God, and told you that God began to play with me more, and make me laugh. We are most of us far too serious about life, and our early images of God were not funny! They were often serious, unfriendly, judgmental—even scary, vindictive and mean. Little did we know back then that those were the mortal qualities of the humans that created that image of God, not of God Itself.

Long before Divine Openings I set a "serious intention" to have more humor in my life. Each time I've asked for this, Life has turned up the laugh track accordingly. Funny friends showed up, funny movies, funny incidents, funny thoughts and scenarios appeared in my mind for my own entertainment. To this day I am unabashedly goofy with friends and in courses.

I transformed my relationship with my worrying, unhappy, and used-to-be-critical mother by setting a clear intention that every time I called her I would make her laugh right off the starting line. I couldn't change her life, but I could impact my relationship with her and make it a highlight in her day. I collected jokes to tell her, and started our phone calls talking in funny voices, like, "Hello Mommy, did you think leaving me at the mall in 1965 would get you off the hook forever? I know where you live!" Or I'd scream "Mommy! Moooooommmmmy!" into her answering machine, and she'd hear me and run laughing to pick up the phone. For some reason calling her Mommy makes her feel good. Brings back her younger days. Everyone just wants to feel better.

When I first started Divine Openings, Mom sat me down and asked me if I was in a cult. I looked at her with horror and retorted, "I can't *believe* you could even *think* I could be such a sheep! I am *not* in a cult—(I paused for comic effect)—I am *leading* a cult!" She nearly fell down laughing and never brought it up again.

Even when my dad was in the hospital a lot, I'd call her and make her laugh. By then she understood (well, at least intellectually) the concept of how important it is to keep your vibration up and only occasionally gave me grief for not being in grief with her!

Most delightfully, my spiritual power has taken a big step forward each time I asked for more humor. Of course, knowing that everything is vibrational, that's no surprise; humor raises your frequency. I've always gravitated to spiritual teachers with a sense of humor, and avoided the dour, pious, over-serious ones. Ugh, if that's what you get from them, I'll pass.

Some years ago I was madly in love with a man who didn't laugh much and didn't get my humor at all. I asked for humor in all my relationships after that, and got it. I wrote about it in my first book, *Dating To Change Your Life* (available at www.DivineOpenings.com.) The next relationship was with a man who was very funny, loved to laugh, totally "got" my humor, and thought I was the funniest person he'd ever met. We laughed daily and had a smooth, carefree, harmonious domestic life that was perfect for that stage of our lives, though it was not a match on the romantic level. There was eventually a parting, and we moved on to more fulfilling partners. I never again dated anyone who didn't have a well-developed, light, and enthusiastic sense of humor.

A romantic partner of mine turned an interview with 2006 Texas gubernatorial candidate Kinky Friedman into a friendship, and one day he took me out to lunch with him to meet Kinky. Kinky is funny as hell but rather deadpan, and is used to being the funny one himself. After observing the man and me together for a bit Kinky inquired, "Is this a serious relationship?" Without missing a beat, I offered, "No, this is a humorous relationship."

That relationship was marked by frequent laughter, and often, it was out of control, wheezing, snorting, belly-aching, side-splitting, donkey-braying laughter. We looked for opportunities to make each other laugh. One day he had just had a Divine Opening and was in my living room standing on his head doing his yoga/karate workout, when he saw the dog's tail bouncing by outside the window. From his upside down viewpoint he thought it was some kind of strange bird hopping by on one wing. He got so broken up when he realized it was the dog's tail that he toppled off his headstand and couldn't get up for laughing.

It's always my intention to look for reasons to laugh. But just as often, reasons to laugh find me. That same friend was poking around checking where he'd left his glasses. He lifted the sleeping dog's butt up and looked under it. Now, I don't know about you, but I had never seen anyone look under a dog's butt for any lost item, and I ripped into convulsions of stomach-cramping giggles, which invariably leads to wheezing, which got us both going even more. Before long, we were both paralyzed and gasping for breath.

Another time, he made a really good omelet with vegetables and avocado. Doing omelets properly had always escaped me. I sleepily said I'd cook next time if he'd "show me how to cook one of those, uh, folded-over things." We were off, laughing uncontrollably, the sounds of our hooting cracking me up even more. I snorted with food in my mouth, then grabbed a napkin to prevent food-spraying, upon which he said, "If you don't watch out, some of that yellow folded stuff with the green filling is going to come out your nose."

So to demonstrate expertly how that could easily be prevented, I stuck the two corners of my napkin up my nose. Then we had a running gag going, and when my long blond hair was in the waffle syrup, he'd say, "Oh, your long yellow stuff is hanging in the sticky stuff." One day he offered, "Here, the feathery red critters made you one of those brown oval things." To that I offered, "There'd be more of those if the long scaly thing wasn't eating them."

When you regain the innocence of a child, there is nothing too silly to do if it will get a laugh, so be generous with your laughter. I remember reading somewhere that polite European society used to deem it unrefined to laugh out loud, and so they suppressed their laughter, allowing only a slight smirk to betray their amusement, lest they look like commoners. There are remnants of that old belief hanging around today, and I am so glad to be free to laugh and show my appreciation and delight. I used to notice in my corporate classes that when people let go of their reserved professionalism and laughed, they really got the material and were more alert, happy and engaged all day.

With very little provocation, just from glancing over and seeing a glint in the other's eye or a hint of a mischievous smile on the other's lips, a Divine Openings Giver and I might rip into uncontrollable spasms. The best was when laughter and joy would overtake us for absolutely no reason; it's called "causeless bliss," and it comes from being up in that high vibration, up in the realms of joy and bliss, where laughter is completely spontaneous and needs no reason. When you're One with The Divine, there is pure joy of being, and when you live close to that vibration all the time, it takes very little to put you over the top. In those moments I truly have no idea why I am laughing—but it feels so good I don't care.

As you become your Divine Self more of the time it will even be easier to stop as an argument begins and inject humor. Humor dissolves anger like nothing else. One friend got angry with me a few times. Once, he was already upset about a work issue and he became defensive at something I said about it. It undoubtedly activated something very old. I saw the fire flash in his eyes as he set his jaw preparing to fight. Something within me twinkled, and I grabbed his shoulders and looked him straight in the eye, and said, "ME FRIEND!" He was startled at first, and then visibly let go. Then we laughed.

When people get caught up in an emotion, especially an old one, logic goes out the window. It's as if a lit match was tossed into a dry haystack. Talking about it logically can go in circles for hours, because it isn't logical. You know this. Humor can fire-hose the whole flame in a few words.

Occasionally, causeless bliss erupts in the Five-Day Silent Retreat. Someone feels a tickle inside and lets it loose, and we all end up hooting like monkeys. Or tears will come that suddenly turn to bliss. You could call it "The Divine laughing you." I feel no need to know why. The need to know the why's in life fade as one just enjoys living.

Every day brings opportunities to laugh if you notice them. Just start reading funny books, watching funny movies, seeking out funny friends. Remember and tell jokes off the Internet, all the while noticing what it is that makes things funny. Note how funny people, and good story and joke tellers, time their punch lines. There's an art to it and you can pick it up; be easy about it. This isn't work, this is joyful play, and there is no deadline. Pattern your delivery after the pros at first, and then you'll develop your own style. Notice the voice tones they use, and how they play the surprise element to get the laugh. Experiment with how long to pause before delivering the zinger, and pay attention to the things other people find funny. The more you laugh, the more Life will match you up with opportunities to laugh, and make others laugh.

So, what a homework assignment this is! To practice laughter and be funnier than ever before! Write this intention in your notebook, and jot down a few ideas for how to have more humor in your life. The Blog and Forum at www.DivineOpenings.com supports you in this.

Develop the gift of humor.

One night as I lay in my bed giving a long distance Divine Opening to my very ill dad, glee bubbled through me from out of nowhere, and I began to chuckle, then to laugh out loud as I felt his spirit soar. It was a great reminder that no matter how grave the illness, how dire the situation looks from our human perspective, The Divine in us experiences joy all the time. Knowing this makes any situation better.

A simple way
to shift your vibration is to ask,
"What is my Large Self feeling right now?"
The answer is always "bliss"
or "everything is fine."

Divine Opening

THIS WORK OF ART is the pure essence of Grace and joy in uncertain circumstances.

Sit quietly and contemplate the image for two minutes.
Then close your eyes and lie down quietly for fifteen or more minutes.

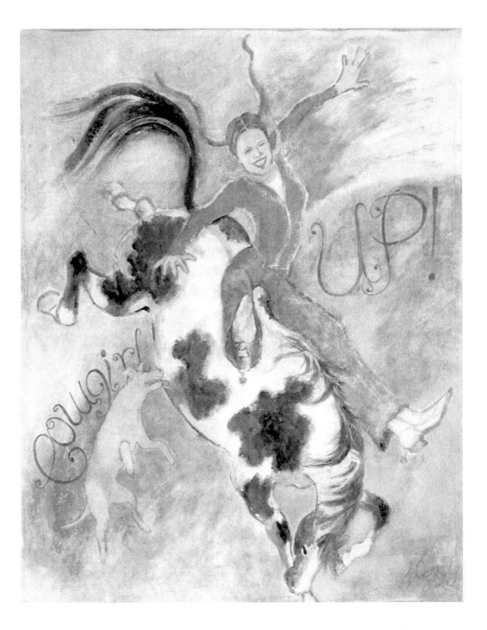

Figure 4 - Cowgirl Up, painting by Lola Jones.

Meditation Made Easy

MEDITATING GETS EASIER with Divine Openings. You can meditate because it feels good—not to be good, be spiritual, or get somewhere (none of that wins you any brownie points or rewards.) Do it to savor your inner silent core and enjoy your expanded self rather than to try to attain some goal. Let go of what other people have told you about their experiences and have your own experience. Deep, sweet feeling is worth as much as all of the mystical visions in the universe.

There is no magic formula, and no single way that is best for everyone. I suggest you follow your heart. I keep it very simple. You don't need rules, gadgets, dogmas or complicated secret rituals. If it's too much work, how can you relax and let The Divine do the heavy lifting?

- Sit or lie quietly in any comfortable position. Close your eyes and focus gently on your breathing. Breathe soft and slow from your belly.

- Now begin to savor your breathing. Notice how wonderful breathing is. Imagine diving down deep into your inner self as you breathe. Think "yes" as you inhale with a tiny smile, and "ah" as you exhale with a slack jaw.

- If thoughts come, don't "follow them." Let them float on by like clouds. Gently return your focus to your breath as many times as you need to. At some point if you get guidance or supportive information, do pay attention, but don't seek it out. Let go.

Meditate for enjoyment, to feel the pure essence that is you.

Morning and Evening "Raves"

FOR OVER A YEAR, each night before I went to bed and when I first woke up, whether I felt great or less than great, I spent a few minutes raving about what I appreciated. By focusing passionately and expressively on what was good in my life and celebrating everything I was happy about, I deliberately raised my vibration. Now it's become a natural habit I do many times a day.

Appreciation is the same vibrational frequency as love. Most humans have some highly charged and distorted concepts about love, and may even find "love" hard to muster when they're not happy with someone. But the concept of appreciation is clear and clean, so it's easier and simpler to call up appreciation than love. Even if you can't conjure love for a person right this now, you can always authentically find something to appreciate about them.

Raving about what's good trains the mind to look for things to love, admire, and appreciate, then more of those vibrations are magnetized to you. We always have the choice of where to put our focus: on what is "wrong"—or what is "right." What is "bad"—or what is "good." What we "like"—or what we "don't like". Make your choice by what feels better, by which feeling or thought brings you more into agreement with your Divine Presence. Does this feel better—or that?

And soon, you find less good/bad duality in your perceptions, it's all considered "experience" and it's easier to feel good in any circumstance. Right now you can choose where to put your focus and feel better in minutes. Today is all that really counts. Yesterday is gone, and tomorrow isn't here yet. Right now is where your power is.

In a recent group Divine Opening, as usual I sat with my eyes closed and evoked a powerful vortex for the group of twenty-seven people, and then everyone sat for a few minutes in the Divine Presence and experienced its effects.

When I asked if a few people would share their experiences, one older woman who was quite experienced on the spiritual path shared a profound experience. She saw scenarios from her whole life appear in front of her. Some events had seemed "bad," and others had seemed "good," and they eventually arranged themselves like a mosaic. Then to her surprise she noticed that all of them now seemed equally OK to her. There was no more sense that some had been good and some bad. It wasn't that they all became "good" so much as that it simply didn't make sense to label them anymore. This is the sign of enlightenment called "equanimity" where, by Grace, you inexplicably accept what is or was, without suffering, without story, and without judgment. It's not just a change in perception—it's a leap to a new dimension of consciousness beyond suffering.

Another way to define equanimity is letting everything be, without resisting it, knowing it's temporary. Everything flows on by—the wanted and the unwanted. And the more freely we let it flow, the more bliss we feel, even in adverse circumstances.

Until appreciation becomes a minute-by-minute habit for you, a morning and evening time of "raving and appreciating" lifts your altitude and your attitude until you naturally reach equanimity, then you are free of the mind and its judgments.

I find it exciting to think that even our wildest dreams of enlightenment and empowerment will pale in the face of what actually comes. We are just beginning to see how we create our reality. In a not-too-distant future, you will literally create worlds, whole realities, for fun. I do.

Make raving a habit.

The Call Of The Divine May Sound Like Success, Sex, or Money

MOST PEOPLE AREN'T consciously seeking enlightenment. I used to notice if I mentioned it in a social setting very few people were interested—they were seeking money, a better relationship, freedom from suffering, world peace, better health, or solutions to problems. These drives for emotional or material desires are fueled by the natural inner drive to feel better, which is the call of The Divine. The Presence within you calls you to feel good and thrive. Although some don't know it, they do want enlightenment. They want restoration to their wholeness, which brings bliss as well as the mundane solutions they seek. Whatever they call it, and however they arrive at enlightenment's door is OK with me.

Relationship, health, inner peace, reduced stress and more money or success are what most people come to me wanting. It's the "big five" that top the list of what most people want and don't have. Their Large Self lures them home with whatever carrot they most want. One woman had already opened up tremendously by her second session with me. Her mind had quieted, and the bouts of anxiety and worry faded or were short-lived. Anger at her kids had calmed.

Her third Divine Openings session was even more profound. She said she wanted a rich man who would take care of her. "OK, you can have that man," I declared with an authority that comes from The Divine within. "Put it on your list of things you want, and in the meantime I have some things for you to consider."

"First, it's all too easy to start thinking that some person, especially some powerful or rich person, is our Source. They are actually just one conduit through which Life sends blessings to us. But what if we get into scarcity, thinking a man is the only place we can get that love or money or care? What if we give our power away to them? Life can bring us what we need through any number of people or circumstances, if we allow it.

"Second, Life brings us more of what we are already feeling. So if you are now feeling a lack of this abundance, and that's why you need this man to take care of you, Law of Attraction can only bring you more lack. If you were to start feeling rich right now, you won't be needy, Law of Attraction can more easily bring you a rich man, you will be a match to his vibration, and so he can stay with you. In America we already are rich as any sultan was two hundred years ago if we just stop and rave about that rather than focusing on what we still don't posess.

"Third, your relationship with The Divine will be reflected outwardly in your romantic relationship. Just for this week, have a love affair with God first. Go directly to Pure Source for the love, the conversation, and the companionship you want—and over time, watch who shows up on the outside. Walk and talk with your Creator, who adores you, loves you exactly as you are, and takes care of you—and can you just imagine who would show up to match that in the physical?"

I evoked a Divine Opening at the end, and went back to my office to write while she rested. After a long rest, tears filled her eyes, and she had difficulty talking without breaking up. She said, "I felt enveloped, hugged, nurtured by The Divine, and then I could feel its Presence sitting next to me, as if waiting to listen, talk to me, whatever I needed. It has filled my empty heart." In that moment, she had moved from lack to fullness.

"Give yourself appreciation for being open to let this gift in," I smiled. "You have opened the door to many blessings." That relationship continued to deepen. In the following week, she had some intense neck pain (probably tension or struggle energy letting go), and her chiropractor's efforts to adjust it didn't help. During sleep that night she saw and felt a physical hand press on her neck, and in the morning the pain was gone. I cannot imagine a better example of how our worldly desires for relationship, material things, health, or relief, are always ultimately calling us back to our relationship with The Presence.

Your Large Self is always calling you home
in whatever way you are most easily enticed.

How The Divine Sees Us

ONE CLIENT HAD a remarkable experience from her first Divine Opening that continued to unfold for her over many months. She sat perched on the sofa in a room with about twelve people. As I evoked the Divine Opening, she immediately saw herself with nine-foot tall white wings. The most remarkable part of her experience was that she saw herself exactly as The Divine sees her, as absolute perfection. She felt it deep in her being. She'd been an exotic dancer once, and had some self-judgment and doubts about her worthiness. Now there was *no* doubt: as she saw every line on her fifty-year-old face in 3-D, lovingly magnified, there was adoration in the gaze. She was The Divine looking at The Divine, and it was One with her. The Divine adores us. It makes no difference what we've done or left undone, no matter who we are or how lost. It is only humans who judge.

Sometimes it's more of a feeling. Others just feel an overwhelming love encompass them, and in that moment they know they are loved. Others feel nothing at all, but good things just happen.

The Divine adores you . . . and IS you.

Unhooking From Ancient Mind

CARL JUNG SPOKE often of the collective consciousness of humanity. Since every thought that has ever been thought is still there, there is a giant pool of collectively shared human vibration you could call Ancient Mind. It is helpful to know that we are much of the time hypnotized by the thoughts and vibrations that we pick up from Ancient Mind, and we buy into a consensus reality that's quite limiting. Remembering that the Ancient Mind can hold others hostage helps me feel compassion for people who are doing horrendous things, because I know that they are not at this time able to access their Large self.

Ancient Mind radiates strong vibrations in the range of fear, scarcity, protection, anger, separation and illusion. It also includes the positive emotions of joy, love and peace as well, but until we are highly conscious and awake, we have little choice as to what vibrations we are picking up from it and acting out. I know how impossible it was for me to unhook from it before Divine Openings shifted my consciousness away from it en masse.

Sometimes it's challenging to escape its pull to find the way to happy, enlightened thinking and actions. Have you ever had a situation where you knew how you wanted to be and act, but couldn't for the life of you do it? We all have. It's like being sucked down into quicksand—wanting to do one thing but to our horror doing something we don't want to do instead. It's as if we've all been plugged into a circuit that charges us up with a discordant energy. When you plug a lamp into the wall, it has no choice about where to get its power. Now we're beginning to plug into a cleaner, purer power source, and the energy we charge up with is different.

Divine Openings unhooks us from Ancient Mind, we plug into pure positive energy, and we begin to vibrate more in harmony with Pure Source.

As we unhook from Ancient Mind, we sometimes experience the dying gasps of its long-practiced patterns. No worries—they're temporary and they pass, leaving you freer than ever each time. As you activate the "positive" energies, the "negative" ones die off from disuse. Literally, as more humans unplug from Ancient Mind, it loses its power. To set our relationships right we must unhook from Ancient Mind, while having compassion for those who are still in its grip. Not just reading but *doing* the upcoming activities in this book frees you from that conditioning.

The Divine Intelligence waking up within each of us is powerful pure consciousness with no limiting consensus reality. We are the many that are One. We came here to experience individuality, and know our oneness—to create individual realities, but not conformity.

Everyday Relationships Are The Key To World Peace

ONENESS WAS MERELY a nice unattainable intellectual concept until I began to have the actual experience of The Divine waking up within me. As the small self lets go, we lose the angst of separateness, competition, danger and scarcity. When we are a part of All That Is, what is there to fear or defend from? We lose our fear of "others" as we realize there are no others. Even though for all practical human purposes I know that my body and my self is separate from yours, I realize we are still part of the same stream of life, we are made of the same stuff, we come from the same Source. I cannot harm the seeming other without literally hurting myself. This is the true beginning of great relationships, where we choose our actions by how it feels rather than how we "should" act.

As more of the inhabitants of this world enlighten, we will easily and spontaneously solve environmental, political, social, and economic crises from a whole new consciousness that sees possibilities we cannot now see. The current state of affairs is the natural product of the current collective consciousness and its consensus reality that limits what's possible. Once our thinking gets more up to speed with the Divine Intelligence within us, we more consistently operate at what is now thought of as genius level. Every person has the seeds of their own unique genius within.

We all have factions within our own selves that disagree or conflict with each other. It is that discord within each of us that manifests out there in the world as conflict and war. When we judge, loath, or criticize ourselves, and resist or reject aspects of ourselves instead of just experiencing them and allowing them to be, there is war within us. When we are disconnected from our Large Self that is always peaceful, there is war within. When there is struggle and unrest with our own families, it is the same energy as war.

Peace begins within each of us, with compassion and acceptance for ourselves—from a quiet, calm mind, allowing of all our parts and aspects. As all our scattered parts are accepted, valued, and experienced, they are soothed—they make peace. Then, from that peaceful and quiet place within ourselves, the love that is our true nature flows from us without trying. The heart flowers. From there it is a natural result to begin to authentically feel and give more love, appreciation, and compassion for our beloveds, families, co-workers, and friends. Then we begin to feel oneness with our city, our country, the world and so on, as this inner peace ripples out into the world. We are each a broadcast station for whatever energy we predominantly generate. Do not underestimate how powerful a generator you are.

Mother Teresa was asked for advice on how to promote world peace.
Her reply was, "Go home and love your family."

The logical extension of the inner peace we gain through Divine Openings is outer peace. Peace doesn't mean agreement. It can mean respectfully agreeing to disagree.

Only from the Large Self can there be genuine relationship with a lover, a child, a parent or a work group. Relationships from small-self-perspective are inauthentic and transactional, guarded, conflicted, conditional, needy, brittle, easily shattered, and lonely. From the Large Self, relationships are unconditional, allowing of differences, rich and deep, safe, rewarding, eternal, and ever expanding. Unconditional love doesn't mean you stay with someone. Unconditional love means you allow someone to *be as they are and as they are not.* You love them no matter how it plays out in the physical. You love them from near or far as you choose.

Fully experience another's perspective, see the world through their eyes and feel the world through their perceptions—and you truly begin to relate. Nelson Mandela says it took him twenty-two years in prison to let go of his anger, see from the perspective of his "enemies," and make them his friends. Only then was he released, to transform his country and its people. He was not a perfect man; you don't have to be perfect to do great good.

Relating is different from relationship. "A relationship" is a thing to control or possess. "Relating" is a process that is allowing, flexible, alive, and active.

Call it a relationship and it is too easily perceived as something set in stone. Life is change, so if a relationship isn't changing, *it's us not letting it.* Fear has us try to control it, preserve, or freeze it. Relate to your mother, your father, your lover in each moment, and it becomes an active process requiring your heart and your full presence. Decide to *experience* (not just conceptualize) true relating in relationship, and giving and receiving become barely distinguishable.

Compassion, love, and oneness cannot be legislated or mandated. How successful have our laws and prisons been at mandating and controlling crime and terrorism? Trying to change people from the outside by controlling people is short term at the very best. Fortunately, there is no need to force, manipulate, or legislate peace. It springs from within each individual authentically as enlightenment flowers—and as more and more individuals know their own Divinity and feel their oneness with everyone else, peace will spread. Enlightened beings naturally make choices and create solutions that reflect their knowing of who they truly are.

From there, getting along with, honoring and collaborating with other families, factions and eventually other countries is a natural flow rather than a figuring out of how-to. There is no other way to act once we know who we are—when we've experienced our whole self, our Large Self.

It starts at home. Your loving peaceful heart creates outer peace in your world.

OK, So How Do I Clean Up My Relationships?

GRACE HELPS YOU and Large Self guides you. Your intention and sincere willingness to get free are all you need. Divine Source is not going to force you to get free against your will. It is your choice, but you don't have to know *how* to do it, you just have to say, *I want it. Do it for me or show me how.* Then The Indweller provides the means and the how to's. Don't make it work. It's not complicated. Your job is just to relax, let go of resistance, and allow it to happen.

In a Houston workshop, in the silence in her own mind after her first Divine Opening, a participant saw, in her mind, a brief slide show featuring her deceased mother, who had not been kind to her. She felt the discord, felt it release, and "knew" it was done. Complete! She came to the workshop with the intention to move her life forward, but she didn't expect to resolve her relationship with her mother. Her Large Self knew how vital it is to clean up key relationships, and Divine Grace did the work. Many clients had a similar "slide show" that provided instant resolution for them, devoid of the dramatic emotion of the original experiences. Some have just *felt something resolve* without knowing or seeing any details. Others hear and feel nothing during the Divine Opening, but then "something happens" in the coming days. One woman's dad called her for the first time in thirty years the day after a Divine Opening. She didn't feel "forgiveness." She felt love.

God Doesn't Forgive!

A WOMAN PRAYED to God fervently for months for forgiveness for some awful things she had done. One night, exhausted from her suffering, she lay in bed and gave up, just hoping to die. Then she heard a voice saying, "I can never forgive you…" She panicked and began to wail. But the voice continued, "…because I never judged you."

The Presence doesn't judge you, punish you, or hold grudges. Humans do. I recently heard that an Amish mother whose child was killed in a school shooting declared that she would hold no grudges. To set an example that others could follow, she purchased thousands of erasers imprinted with the words "grudge eraser" and gave them away at media events.

People spontaneously open their hearts without effort to people they had shut out, sometimes after having a single Divine Opening. In the instant their perspective shifts to Large Self they wonder why it was so difficult or complicated to just let it go. Once that shift occurs, the word "forgiveness" doesn't begin to describe what happens. From that new consciousness, there is never anything to forgive, because your Large Self never judged in the first place.

After a Divine Opening, one woman was guided from within to list about ten people she'd been "trying to forgive" for years, and as she went down the list, one by one intending to "work on it"— she noticed there was nothing left to forgive! All that remained was peace and even love.

Think about it. Doesn't it sound a bit arrogant to say to someone, "I forgive you"? As if your small self ever held the right to judge them? And now you deign to say they're OK? I think of it now as "letting go" or "freeing myself." It's me choosing to return to Large Self perspective. I had been carrying that anvil; now I put it down. I had been nursing that pain; now I walk on, a free woman.

It feels more accurate to me to say, "I've stopped judging you," than to say, "I forgive you."

Rather than saying, "I forgive you,"
try this: "I've stopped judging you."

I say to them in my own mind, "I know your inner Divinity and your worthiness." Letting go of hurts you've been clinging to *frees you* and stops the poisoning of your body and soul from resentment, anger, and sadness. That's the best reason to do it. Not for them.

The only good use I've found for the word forgiveness is to forgive *myself*. Judging or condemning yourself is the most damaging thing you can do in all of creation.

Say to yourself, "I forgive you for creating this. I love you."

Releasing Past Hurts

SIT QUIETLY and speak inside your heart to anyone who has hurt you, living or dead. Tell them how you felt, and what you wanted from them. Don't go over the story. Just how you felt and what you wanted. Period. "I felt worthless when _____ happened. I wanted to feel valued and loved."

One man went into the stillness inside and asked The Presence to be with him as he told his deceased father how hurt he had been when his father had beat him from childhood up to his teen years. He told his father that he had wanted to be hugged and praised. Love flooded him as he was freed from that burden, and as he felt how tortured his father had been.

Once you've done this, you will know if you need to say something to the real live person. And if you do speak to them, say it from the perspective of how you felt and what you wanted, rather than making it about what they did. Let go of their response. This is for your freedom.

Free Yourself, The Rest Will Follow

IF SOMEONE hurt you in the past, however painful it was, it is now history. You are learning how to attract something better in the future. Experience the emotion without the story, your vibration rises, and you are free. If you remain a victim and keep regenerating that emotion and vibration by telling and retelling the terrible story to yourself and others, now who's hurting you? You are hurting yourself over and over by continuing to hold onto that feeling.

It's too difficult to try to figure out logically who hurt whom first, and why. The chain of pain passes down through thousands of generations—people who hurt you were themselves in pain of some kind, and so it goes, back into ancient history. But with ease and Grace it can end with you now. When you free yourself, it ripples out to humanity.

You think you wanted others to be there for you, but what you really needed was to be there for yourself. Start being there for yourself right now, like a big brother or sister, even if no one else was there for you back then. This incredibly powerful decision changes your past, present, and future, and most importantly, it allows The Presence to be there fully for you.

Even if that other person wasn't there for you, now YOU are there for you.

You are the only one you have any control over. Make the decision to let go, and let The Divine do the heavy lifting. Ask to know Truth, to know Oneness, to allow Life Source to flow fully through you. Ask for any obstacles to be moved. Working on it adds resistance to resistance so intend that this process occur for you with ease and grace. Experience, embrace, and breathe into that feeling without thinking about it, and let it rise and resolve.

It's *your love* that's been shut off, and when you let it flow again, you are liberated, restored to your true Self. Do it for you, not for the other person. If your love pipeline stays closed, your life energy is pinched off, you contract, and you are out of alignment with your Large Self. Your Large Self never has to forgive, because your Large Self never judges. The only person it makes any sense to forgive is you. You might say, "I forgive myself for creating that reality."

Relationships are what life in this dimension is about, and they are one of the keys to your freedom. By letting go of hurts, you are *not* saying it was OK—you are saying that you choose being happy over being right. You are claiming your power to free yourself. As you practice being there for yourself, you find your Large Self was already there, waiting for you, calling you to freedom. As you get back in alignment with your Large Self, everything looks and feels different.

The chain of pain can end with you.
You are free when you let go.

With compassion (not judgment) I tell you these next two stories, to make the point that even with the blissful free rides Grace gives, we must sustain our enlightenment and bring it down to earth. The *conscious mind piece* of Divine Openings is only about ten percent of the total, but it is necessary for our awakening. Remember the friend I mentioned who, before we met, had a very flashy cosmic oneness experience you might think would be anyone's ultimate, end-all bonanza? She was in orgasmic ecstasy for months, but it may surprise you that once it was over, her life didn't change much. She did get contented living simply on little money, but she still holds family grudges, justifies it, doesn't believe she creates her reality, is accident-prone (matching the belief that problems in her life are accidental), and although she is gorgeous and sexy, lovers don't stay. She still reads literally hundreds of spiritual books, but still isn't willing to feel lower vibrations and claim authorship of her life.

"Energy junkies" chase the cosmic energy highs, but try to avoid ordinary feelings, denying they create them, or blaming them on others.

A PhD psychologist who didn't read this book had a spontaneous cosmic explosion of ecstasy and oneness that lasted weeks, long before we met. Afterward, he went back to resenting ex-spouses, continued attracting heartbreaks, and teaches Law Of Attraction but struggles with living it. The awakening is permanent only when we do our part to bring it "down to earth."

Grace tosses you aloft like a dove into flight. Your conscious choices keep you there.

This activity, along with the Divine Opening that follows, frees you and restores your flow. Your job is simply to get out of the way and allow it to happen—to be willing. *There's no work to do.* In your notebook, make a list of people in your life, past and present, living and dead, where love is even a wee bit withheld by you, or where your love is not fully flowing.

The key relationships are parents, siblings, children, family members, spouses, ex-spouses and partners.

Next are business associates and friends.

Include yourself—is love fully flowing for yourself? Do you adore yourself as The Divine does?

How about government leaders, your president, politicians?

Enemies of your nation? Terrorists? People who pollute the environment?

People at work? Rich, greedy people? Poor, lazy people?

People who are closed-minded, mean, perverted?

People who put other people down?

Those who let you down, broke your heart, or you broke theirs.

People who clearly did you wrong.

Ones where you're on the good guys' side and they're clearly (really!) the bad guys.

Anyone who hooks you, or that you have an emotional charge on.

If your list is blank and your love flows freely to everyone on the planet, first check if you're being honest! If it's true, sit and enjoy letting this unconditional love radiate from you. Your intention might be, "How do I go deeper?" or, "Make me a beacon."

Remember: all the people on your list have been in the grip of Ancient Mind, just as you were, and their thoughts and "choices" were often not their own. Remember they too wanted to feel and act better, and be free of the bondage to their mind and emotions. But they could not, just as you could not always do it. Ask your Large Self for help in raising vibration about relationships so that you may be liberated and your enlightenment can fully flower. You don't have to do the work, just be willing to turn it over to The Indweller, and it's all taken care of.

ACTIVITY: Stop reading and do this now. Reading doesn't make it happen:

Place your hand over your heart.

Let it be the hand of your Large Self, The Indweller, The Divine Presence.

Whisper your hurts, disappointments, losses.

Express *what you wanted that you didn't get.*

Let The Divine raise any lower vibrations in you to higher ones.

Intend your heart to open, and to let go of pain and resistance.

Receive the next Divine Opening on the coming page.

(On a separate occasion do this for all those *you have hurt*.)

Note in your journal over the next few days or weeks what you notice about your relationships. You may have felt nothing extraordinary in the activity and Divine Opening, yet relationships open up by themselves, love flows, or you just feel better about it. Celebrate any movement.

Advanced Perspective

FROM YOUR LARGE SELF perspective you recognize that you create your reality. Moving all the lower emotions as you feel them helps you authentically rise up out of them. Don't be "responsible for your reality" in a small-self, victim-like way. Be kind to yourself. Get your vibration up before you take too much responsibility. Take your power back first.

From Large Self, declare, "I created that," and feel your power swell. You don't need to know why you created it. The answer will come if you need to know.

Don't analyze, push yourself, or struggle with this. It may be that upon the third or fourth reading of the book, this will suddenly seem natural and effortless. You can celebrate that day when it comes!

There is no hurry. Your Large Self patiently calls to you, yet judges you not.

When you own that you created it, you get your power back.

This book, at Level One, is primarily about getting free from suffering and into peace or joy; getting your Large Self in the front seat more of the time. Divine Openings is not about speed bumps and hairballs forever. If you're still struggling, you can be absolutely sure Grace is doing its part; but you must use your Free Will to do your part. Are you still listening to your mind's scary stories? Are you doing the activities instead of just reading?

A couple of times I've gone into in-your-face-cowgirl-guru mode and said to a client, "*Make a decision!* Get mad if you need to! Decide to stop letting your mind run your life. No more of that! *Decide now* to keep the nose tipped up, and decide that nothing—*nothing*—is worth tipping the nose of your plane down for long! This is your precious life. *Only you* can make this choice. I can't make it for you. You have Free Will." They got the wake-up call, made their choice, and it took them to a whole new level.

To reinforce your new choices or to accelerate your progress, you may enjoy taking the Level One Self-Paced Online Retreat. It includes videos and scores of audio recordings of one-to-one sessions and voluminous material that came through after this book was written. As I'm channeling during those sessions, the Energy is thrilling enough, but what comes through me in answer to clients' specific needs and desires on every topic is astounding (and sometimes amusing.) Make choices that nourish and support you, in every way, in every part of your life. Most important, choose to enjoy life right now—that's more powerful than getting "more advanced."

Divine Opening

THIS WORK OF ART activates a specific Energy/Light/Intelligence. Many people reported spontaneous physical healings from this particular piece. It is one of my personal favorites; the originals all hang in my home. Sit quietly, and contemplate the image for two minutes. Then close your eyes, lie down, and savor for fifteen minutes or longer.

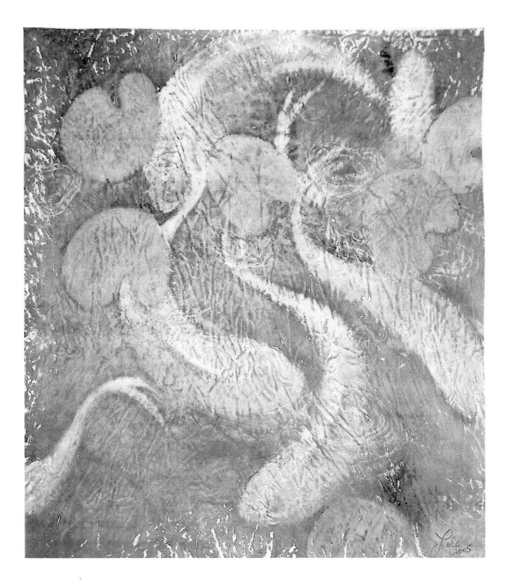

Figure 5—Goldfish, painting by Lola Jones

Romantic Relationships

IT'S AMAZING WHAT love feels like when you're free, fulfilled, and whole. Oneness with your own Large Self gives security and stability regardless of your outer life, and regardless of who does or doesn't love you. This increases your ability to experience love for another person instead of the illusion of them or the need of them. A togetherness that might have seemed excessive or co-dependent in the old paradigm becomes normal and healthy in the new one because it is between two people who know who they are and are in their own center.

Sex is amazing when you feel what your partner is feeling and thrill to it—when you stroke their skin and feel your own pleasure increase. When love circulates in an intimate loop, pleasure increases terrifically. It's a beautiful aspect of our oneness. By the same token, if you hurt someone, you feel it. When you know that the other is "You," you cannot hurt them without experiencing pain, and you can't give pleasure without experiencing it yourself. Fights don't happen often when communication is simple, direct, and kind.

When the sense of separation between two people is diminished and they realize they are the male and female counterparts of each other (in heterosexual couples, at least, which is all I know about) the intimacy becomes so much sweeter. You can look at your partner with delight, seeing a fascinating masculine or feminine mirror of yourself.

It is easy to truly care for another when you know them as yourself and as an expression of The Divine. Deeper connectedness in sex goes far beyond physical sensation and friction, and even far beyond love. Lovemaking is a door to higher consciousness when the heart is open. Just as there is no ceiling to human evolution, there is no ceiling to love and intimacy.

Relationship becomes a whole new experience when your relationship with yourself is already strong and supportive—when there is no neediness, no emptiness to fill, no lack to try to escape. The black hole of neediness attracts more lack of love. When you feel full, you attract more love, and your relationship experiences are easier. The painful, aching, longing feeling many people associate with love is actually the feeling of the absence of love or the awful fear of losing it.

Relationship problems dissolve quickly when one can be with the emotions that arise and flow through the self and the beloved—when one experiences emotion without identifying with it, and doesn't get swept up in it or the story. When one accepts the other person exactly as they are, suffering ceases. And when your lover feels your genuine self-generated happiness, the burden is off them to be the source of your happiness. What a relief. Then you can play like children.

I have never, however, insisted that romantic relationship must last forever. After two wonderful years, one love and I began to pull in different directions. We were no longer the romantic vibrational match we once were. I felt a deep need to be alone more. I am essentially a free spirit, and found the amount of togetherness he needed stifling. For a while, as friends, we still created outrageously fun and innovative ideas, until he had to stop seeing me so he could move on. Every relationship I've had has been more wonderful than the last.

Relationship for me has been more about evolution than finding the one Mr. Right. I have lived so many lives in this body—I can't imagine who could have handled all those incarnations of me. It makes most people's heads spin. I love them all to this day—real love doesn't end when the relationship changes. Even if you want to be with someone for life, love lightly, and let it unfold naturally. Let it be however it is. If it's to be for life, it will be. You couldn't possibly stop it.

I did feel that there would eventually be one who would fly with me, evolving long term together, at the same pace. I've joked, "While I've never promised till death do us part, one day I'll have that experience, because we'll be so old at least one of us will depart the planet!" I enjoyed life and happily savored the waiting until my love Russell showed up, and I do believe he's that man. Russell and I created a new online retreat to add to your joy: *The Art Of Love and Sex*. We do live life consciously, deliberately, creatively, and playfully, like a daily work of art.

Unconditional Love: A Practical Definition

EVEN BEFORE DIVINE OPENINGS I never understood how people "stop loving" someone after a divorce, breakup, or disagreement. They cut off the flow of their own love, which cuts off part of the flow of their own Life Force. It literally distances them from their Large Self.

Conditional love says "You must please me to get my love." Unconditional love says, "*I am happy no matter how you are.*" You thought I was going to say "I will love you no matter how you are." No, you don't have to *like* what they do, but when you are happy and being your Large Self, *you just love*, because the Large Self is love! Real love doesn't go away when the beloved leaves you or changes. If it goes away, it wasn't really love—it was addiction, or a filler for your emptiness, or possession, or entertainment. True love remains, even if you choose not to live with that person, or they choose not to live with you.

You won't have to work at all this once the Divine Openings have worked on you for a while. Divine Grace allows us to do in minutes what we've struggled with for years. Grace can do for us what we have not been able to do for ourselves. The definition of Grace is a gift you did not earn.

But until you have fully become your Divine Self, constantly refocus your thoughts on what is good in your partner. What you focus on increases. If you focus on what you appreciate about them, you will get more of that. If you focus on what is wrong with them, you will get more of that. Choose wisely. If you find yourself dwelling on their faults, take a minute or so every day to list their good points. Remember how you adored them when you first met? It's the same person after all. Only your focus has changed. The mind, wrong-seeking missile that it is, delights in finding what is wrong. Your Large Self sees only what is right and what could be.

After receiving Divine Openings for a while, one man was delighted that his thirty year relationship with his wife flowered into happiness again after many stalemated years, as he suddenly became aware he had been passively aggressive while appearing nice and cooperative. The old habit was gone and he experienced pure love for his wife again. As the negativity that is not You rises in vibration, love is what's left of You.

It is possible that you and your love will find yourselves out of vibrational alignment at some point, and that you wish to evolve in different ways, or that one chooses to stay in the same vibration while the other wishes to expand. In that case, you can part with love, blaming no one.

Keep your own love pipes open as you part—if you shut any of your love off, your flow is constricted, not theirs. Feel it fully, even if it hurts, and stay open. It will pass, and when your pipes are open and flowing, you're free and energized.

Since there is no sense of scarcity when one is in the flow of All That Is and one with Life, relationships can flow in and out of your life, and you feel no more than a fleeting sense of loss, knowing that you will always have the love you want, both within and outside of you.

Love never ends.

Processes For Transformation

THIS BOOK CONTAINS many processes to help you realign with and live as your Large Self, which naturally leads to all the good things you want in your life. For quick daily reference, at the back of the book you'll find Thirty Ways To Raise Your Altitude (your vibration) and some maintenance practices to keep your altitude high and steady. In every "now" moment, with every thought and feeling, you are creating your tomorrows. All it takes is paying attention and choosing. Relax. You have time to change any lower vibrational thought or feeling before it manifests.

Post a copy of that list where you'll see it often, practice every day, and build new habits. Fortunately it feels so good to do every one of those things, it's play, not work.

Prostrating To The Divine

HERE IS A DETAILED "how-to" on one of the most powerful processes in the book. Photographs illustrate it at www.DivineOpenings.com on the Ask Lola page. Scroll way down.

During my twenty-one days of silence I discovered the beauty of prostrating, and when I got home I used it on those occasions when I wanted to powerfully and clearly give something over to The Divine. It was my silver bullet. You can also prostrate for the pure pleasure of it, out of desire to further relax into Divine Order. I prostrate, not in a pious attitude, because piousness is not authentic for me, and "I am unworthy" is a very low vibration. I do it in the spirit of having my small self let go to my Large Self, to become more blissfully aligned with God, and so dance through life with more ease. Best of all, do it because it feels good!

Before you prostrate you might speak to your Large Self about what you intend, ask for what you need, relax your mind, and get in your feelings. Or you might make a list of all the things you must do or accomplish, and turn it over to The Divine to do for you. The Presence already knows what you want. Prostrating physically demonstrates you're ready to let go and let Grace do it!

Ask for help releasing hurts and restoring love to relationships. Express your intention to let go of being right, working hard, and doing it all yourself. Prostrate to know wisdom, release resistance, get liberation from suffering—whatever you want. This ritual helps unhook you from Ancient Mind and you become a force for the enlightenment of the planet.

There is nothing magic about any ritual—they can focus energy in a powerful way, but don't give them your power. They simply help your mind and body let go. Change the prostrating ritual in any way you desire.

Prostrating Basics:

- Write or speak to yourself about what you want help with, and hold your intent in your mind, or you could put your hand on your heart, or put your hands in a praying position—whatever feels right for you.

- Sit quietly—feel your full feelings and drop the story.

- Prostrate on the floor. Lie face down, body stretched out full length, with your forehead to the floor, your arms stretched out in front of your head with palms together, as in praying position. You can lie on your side, kneel, sit, or do it however you like.

- Lay it all down. Let go. Stop thinking and trying to solve it and just feel.

- Breathe deeply, in big sighs, "for pleasure."

- As you exhale, let it all go, intending your burdens be released to The Presence. Feel the relief when your body gives a final deep sigh.

- Ask to be filled with the feeling and knowing of You as Divine Presence.

Where you are is where you are. You can go anywhere from here.

Sickness and Health

IN THE TWENTY-ONE days of silence, about eighty percent of the people experienced the dissolution of old patterns, childhood conditioning, and other negativity as *sickness* rather than feeling the emotions directly. I didn't experience any sickness because I was willing to be with feelings and move it all emotionally. If one fears lower emotions or thinks that makes them less spiritual, they often try to do the spiritual bypass and mentally gloss over the lower feelings. It doesn't work.

Back at home, one client had repeated accidents as he resisted feelings and avoided claiming he creates it all. Accidents are caused by believing life is random and accidental, or they're a mirror of making choices that hurt oneself. Physical manifestations are the hard way to discover the lower energies if the person won't feel. Some people actually like intense physical symptoms, because they need a sure sign that something powerful is moving.

Masses of lower energy move up with Divine Openings. This is rapid, en mass movement, not the never-ending, bit-by-bit, old-paradigm process that takes a long time. If "all hell breaks loose" when you make a powerful decision to let go of your baggage, that tells you it was *way overdue.* The good news is that it passes quickly if you don't make it wrong or resist what's happening. Some move it with emotional discharge, others with physical discharge or sickness, others by seeing it in the mirror of life. Some people let it move without fanfare; with no resistance, and with total ease.

Anything moving is a good sign. The higher you ascend in altitude, the greater the necessity to jettison any density. As that density rises to higher vibrations, it may be effortless, or it may take the form of discomfort, illness, low emotions, fatigue or dis-ease. I don't even like to call out the names of dis-eases, because then they become a big "thing." Thought, emotion, matter, Spirit—it is all just vibration at different densities. A dis-ease is a vibrational condition; it's not really a "thing" until we name it, diagnose it, focus on it, and make it so. It can be interrupted at any level. Divine Openings interrupts it at a very high spiritual, vibrational level, and then the body reorganizes and restructures. Again, don't resist—choose ease.

We're understandably very concerned about our bodies, but don't get alarmed by a medical diagnosis. Feel it and it can pass easily, or you'll let it resolve in some way, even if you let in medical help. Physical diagnoses of dis-ease are some of the hardest things for people to relax about. When a doctor is saying you have a dis-ease and shows you a chart with evidence, it takes intention, clarity, and focus to disregard that authoritative proclamation and hold to your desired image of health until your vision overpowers the temporary reality of the disease. Stop giving so much *respect* to any unwanted reality—it's all temporary unless you keep giving it reality.

Most of us think we only *observe* reality. But observing it is *creating* it. We observe what is, and vibrate what is, which creates more of what is. Then we observe what is, vibrate what is, and create more of what is. The only reason any reality exists is that you vibrated its essence long enough. For example, when a person vibrates insecurity or concern, stress or anger for long enough, it can eventually manifest as a dis-ease. The well-being that constantly flows keeps you healthy and corrects problems. Resisting the flow is the only reason for dis-ease.

First, accept where you are and relax about it. Release resistance to where you are. Stop observing/creating what is, and turn your powerful attention to what you do want. Then you begin to let in what you want. Then as you observe the improved situation, you let in more improvement.

If you are dealing with physical illness or pain and cannot get relief from using the book, there is more specific help tailored to you in one-to-one sessions and courses. We can often, through our experience and training, see your blind spots easily, where you cannot as yet see them. See www.DivineOpenings.com. We have powerful physical healers listed in the Divine Openings Givers Directory. There are no limits to what can be healed. None. Do always follow your own guidance and get any help you need, including medical. Life offers many options.

Disrespect reality!

Who Are We?

YOU'RE NOT SOME inferior being here to earn your way to some reward, or even worthiness. You are magnificent—the Divine's finest creation, pioneering expansion in the physical dimension. This wondrous world of tastes, smells, light, sound, and touch needs to be tasted by your lips, smelled by your nose, and seen with your eyes. Life enjoys living through us, and it's our choice whether we enjoy it or not! There is great celebration in the non-physical realms when we do.

For millennia, Life has evolved us as a species, developing and preparing our minds and bodies to embody more of The Presence. But new energies coming to the planet now are catalyzing quantum leaps for us by pure Grace, as we prepare for the full descent of Spirit into matter (or you could see it as matter ascending into light.) You may call the awakening whatever you like; the

Mystery cannot be explained by the mind, but it can easily be enjoyed.

The Grace that Divine Openings opens you to gives the brain increasing capability to sustain the higher states and directly experience reality so that we can walk the Earth knowing ourselves as aspects of God. Our physical bodies are evolving to fully embody it long-term.

The Essence Of Life always remains in its vast, formless, multi-dimensional, timeless, non-physical state, but it focuses aspects of itself into many physical forms, including beings like us. Our bodies and the physical things we create are fleeting manifestations, but our Essence continues on through it all, evolving in Intelligence and Wisdom backwards and forwards in time.

There's no risk for an eternal being, since there is no death; there is only life and more life. It was such a freedom when a near death experience showed me I really was not afraid to die! I was actually debating, "Go? Or stay?" with no attachment to the outcome. Now I have years of always being able to reliably find that still, steady, unshakable center inside me that is always steady, no matter what is happening outside. All I do now is tune in, and get myself to the party. Anytime you stop and be still you can find it. Set aside time every day to tune in, whether in meditation, moments of silence, or nature walks.

It became increasingly clear it was always there inside anytime I wanted to experience it. I'd known this as a mental concept for years, but now it was vividly real. Adventures await you on this Earth and within, and your capacities continue to increase astoundingly. You're just beginning to tap in, and the more you do, the more you discover your unused gifts and capacities.

While it may not always be obvious from our small-self perspective, from Larger perspective, we are the early astronauts, braving the unknown to satisfy an inexplicable need to expand our world beyond the prescribed limitations of the old order. Like their Command Central Ground Control, our Universal Intelligence acts as a navigational base system for us, giving us all the support we need to do anything successfully. Our job is to keep our vibration high enough to receive and interpret it accurately, sort of like keeping our satellite dish pointed toward that steady home signal rather than pointing away at some discordant distraction. We're evolving away from the judgment and the suffering caused by the mind's domination. We don't have to know how to do it. Our desire births solutions in the vast Unlimited Intelligence, and we take steps as guided.

It is, after all, our physical selves that expand the physical world, by experimenting in the duality and contrast of the wanted and the unwanted, the "good" and the "bad," while the Essence Of Life remains reliable, blissful, and non-dual. Remember, when you're feeling strong desire for something that isn't manifested yet, it's there for you. If you vibrate in harmony with that desire, you get to experience the joy of it right now, and then it's a bonus that as you vibrate it consistently, something materializes to match it. Even if you don't manage to see it happen in your lifetime, you created it, and contributed it to the evolution of this and all other dimensions. Imagine those science fiction writers like Jules Verne who didn't get to see their stories become reality in this lifetime—they get to experience it in the next. Your desire is never lost or wasted, but waits for you in some other body, place, or time. What we'll evolve into next is beyond imagination. You'll take with you all of your expansion, and go beyond even that. Just imagine it, for fun…

Leading The Universe's Expansion

THE CREATOR HASN'T laid out a plan for all eternity. Creation is ever new, always experimental, always expanding. There's no master plan all finished, waiting for us to figure it out and get it right. There's no test to pass, no wings to earn, no cut to make. There is nowhere to get to because there is no finish line, but you get to do with this life whatever you choose. You are free.

The universe is one eternal, ecstatic explosion of creativity, and we reflect its thirst for experience with more than six billion faces. If you're reading this, chances are that you are one who doesn't follow the norm; you create new possibilities. You're not interested in the status quo. You understand it's all in Divine Order and there's never anything "wrong," but you always want more and better. We're not the cosmic couch potatoes, we're members of a Divine scouting party out on the leading edge of endless creation. Like all explorers, on some level we liked the idea that we'd come to this far-flung frontier where we'd blaze new trails, take risks, try new things, sometimes fail, to get up and try again. You're going to do great things, lightly, easily, breezily.

Ever wonder why you sometimes don't get clear guidance about what to do? It's because you as Divine Presence in a physical body get to create your own directions, inspired ideas, and solutions. You get to try new things, and it doesn't really matter how it works out. There's really no risk in the end because there is no end. You can't fail because it's never over. Of course you want to succeed at endeavors, but soothing yourself this way can help you lighten up and go for it. What do you have to lose? There is guidance, there is that stable base station that has the broader view, with its radar, navigating devices and powerful resources to help, but on this frontier there is no map, only historical evidence, which we're not interested in anyway. We don't want to repeat history; we have bigger desires. Even if it's safer, it's not satisfying. We will continue our exploration of the far fringes of possibility for all eternity, and some of us will come back again and again to this fascinating and yet maddeningly dense and slow (compared to the lightning speed of the non-physical planes) physical environment, into the uncertainty of leading edge pioneering.

The Creator is not complete, finished, and perfect waiting for us "defective ones" to get it right, redeem ourselves, cleanse ourselves, or be good so we get rewarded. We are the Creator's adored physical extensions, bringing this physical dimension more into alignment with the spiritual dimensions, just by being joyful, loving, and creative. Isn't it a relief that it isn't work? Heaven on Earth was here all along; it just takes awakened eyes to see it.

Heaven is right here on Earth.

What Is Enlightenment?

ENLIGHTENMENT IS NO big deal. It is simply returning to the natural state you were designed to live in. You are designed to be happy, healthy, loving, expanding creatures. When you are living in that state all the time it just feels normal. Granted, when you first feel the full surge of Life Force flowing through you, it may feel like you've stuck your toe in a light socket. But when you get accustomed to it, it will feel like no big deal. It is your natural state. A magnificent, healthy, vital racehorse feels good in its body, and it is a miracle to watch, but it is not supernatural. *It is natural.*

If you expect something supernatural, you may be disappointed if that's not your Large Self's path for you. Sometimes that doesn't happen immediately but it opens up over time. Sometimes people who did not ask for supernatural manifestations get them! Let The Divine decide. Can you let go and enjoy whatever wonderful gifts come? If so, they come faster.

Before we dwell on what enlightenment is, I encourage you to relax about the timing and details. You may or may not experience the "classical" enlightenment. Yours will be unique. As enlightenment flowers, you begin to see, feel and experience things that were there all along, but you were unable to tune into. Love for an estranged parent or ex-spouse, a personal relationship with The Divine, appreciation for the beauty in everything—these things were there all along. By Grace, a change inside you suddenly makes it possible to perceive subtleties you couldn't before—mysteriously your AM radio is replaced with an FM radio and now you can get those stations that existed all along, but simply could not be found on your old AM radio dial.

You are literally being hooked up to a rich, complex world wide web, and you don't have to know how it works to enjoy the miracle of it. You don't have to know how a computer works, what makes your heart beat, or how the plants you eat grow to appreciate and benefit from them. As you rediscover your oneness with the unified field, you are once again in harmony with The Essence Of Life that orchestrates everything. When you live consciously as your Large Self, you are led where you need to be; synchronicity has you rendezvous easily with the perfect people for mutual benefit and mutual joy. You know that well-being enfolds you.

Becoming enlightened is a process that definitely has a moment of birth. Divine Openings causes it. There's a crossing of a threshold, and yet it is never quite "finished." If you ask an enlightened being, "Are you enlightened?" the answer is something to the effect of, "I am still evolving, just as everything is still evolving, expanding, and becoming." One who is enlightened has no need to say so. One who has a need to say so is not yet enlightened.

For some, the flowering of enlightenment begins to happen within a few days. For most it is a more gradual process that allows one to acclimate to a wholly new world. My own process was more gradual, unfolding over months, and years, and it is still deepening. I think The Divine gave me a more gradual process so that I could remain in a normal life, relate easily with regular people, and they can relate to me in my imperfection. I help soothe the fears of their small selves, and help them release resistance from a place of having been through it all myself, rather than receiving it in one flash of illumination. The big cosmic flashes aren't the silver bullets you might imagine them to be.

Slow down and savor each day! Slower is often faster.

We are Life Energy in human form, playing in its own creation. When I first saw who I really am, my small self was afraid of the light of my own Being. Your mind may continue to deny that enlightenment has begun to flower and try to continue its old routine. A fan continues to turn even after you turn off the switch. It will slow and stop after a while.

As consciousness expands, we gain conscious access to a broader perspective, and that is what I call "being my Large Self." The Large Self is more wise, loving and powerful than the narrowly focused small self. The small self doesn't need to know all the details when it follows the guidance from the Large Self at Command Central. Astronauts don't need to know every instrument reading that NASA is seeing from the ground; they get the information they need in the moment, to get where they want to go, or to do the job at hand. Your small self is the astronaut; your Large Self is Command Central.

The Supreme Creator, spanning many Universes, many dimensions, and many realities, with its perspective so broad, so vast that we cannot conceive of it, decided to express a small part of itself as a focal point in you, so you are a somewhat narrowed focus of it. The vastly Larger part of you is beyond the physical realm, but you have access to it. Now you can walk the planet as that Large Self, playing this game we call "life on planet Earth" in full mastery. Enlightenment is becoming conscious again of that Larger You. Enlightenment is about waking up to all of who you are. It's about having full access to the Large Self's resources, the greatest of which are love and joy.

Enlightenment is becoming conscious.

Classic Signs of Enlightenment

YOU WILL BEGIN to experience signs of enlightenment and may wonder what to expect or what it all means. The earliest signs of enlightenment are usually increased inner peace, a quieter mind, moments of causeless bliss, and mysterious disappearance of anxiety. Synchronicity amps up. Once you relax into the flow of life, its natural orchestration brings people, circumstances and events together to provide what's needed for all. Life is all connected, all intelligent, all one, so of course it works in concert with your needs and desires. Science calls it the unified field. I asked for a very functional, grounded, connected, practical form of enlightenment, as I wanted to be fully engaged with the world and its business. Some want to sit in a cave somewhere and beam enlightened energy to the world from a distance. That's a worthy service—if it's what you want. I wanted a practical, grounded, spiritual but non-religious, and fun enlightenment. I wanted it to make me even more effective in my business affairs and more loving and available in relationships. You can design your enlightenment just about any way you want to, and later in the book you'll get help doing that.

While there are some classic signs, your enlightenment is unique and not everyone experiences the "classic" variety. These signs may not all appear at once, but as part of an unfolding.

1. Witnessing yourself: Observing yourself objectively from your Large Self, as if from outside yourself, is one hallmark. This "witnessing" of yourself may occur as an actual out-of-body experience where you look down upon your body. It may be a subtle dual perspective, with your wiser, objective Large Self noticing the actions and responses of your more limited small self. That's how I witness. You begin to see the workings of your own mind with clarity and objectivity—not judging, but simply being aware, for example, of the small-self mind's pettiness or defensiveness. Suddenly you see clearly the old habits and beliefs that have ruled your life. The mind may not entirely stop doing what it does, but it no longer controls you. You start to understand that you're not your mind. "Just because my mind says something doesn't mean I have to listen!"

You become less and less identified with or caught up in the dramas, stories and deceptions of the mind as you identify with the Larger Self view. You don't stop being human and fallible, but you are conscious. You are aware of what you are feeling, saying, or doing, and are not run by it. Now I can reach deep states of meditation even when my mind is chattering away. I can just ignore it. I can be productive no matter how I feel. Feelings don't rule me.

2. Equanimity and the end of suffering: The ability to fully experience each moment as it comes your way, without suffering, is "equanimity." This aspect of enlightenment allows a person to experience their current current physical reality, other people, and their own emotions as they are, without resistance to them. The enlightened one appreciates and accepts everything as it is, at peace in the calm at the eye of the storm. Experiences move by in a kaleidoscopic parade. There is less story added to the experience, less dramatizing of the situation. They often say, "It is what it is," or "How interesting that I created *that*," or "Everything is temporary."

Enlightenment has been called the end of suffering. I had a dear friend who was fifty-six, in a nursing home, bedridden, dependent on dialysis, on disability income, and lost both legs from diabetes. I gave him Divine Openings over many months. He went through a deep dark night of the soul at one point, diving to the depths of despair. He left his body and communed with dead relatives in a vast white space with no floor or walls. Then he emerged peaceful and joyful. By the time he passed, he was one of the happiest people I knew. He uplifted the doctors and nurses. Even though his body was diminished and he could not reverse it, he did not feel powerless. He was hopeful. He was enlightened.

My personal experience has been a gradual diminishment, then loss of the ability to suffer— literally to the point where very little disturbs my inner peace for longer than a few minutes, or at the very worst, a few hours or a day. When we experience things from Large Self perspective, or God perspective, there is nothing to suffer about. Even if someone dies, we know there is no real death, just a change of form. If we lose something or someone, we know that there is no scarcity. When we look at suffering in the world, we hold the energy of the solution, and we know that's more powerful than suffering over their suffering, which only adds to the vibration of suffering and creates more of it in us and out there. Don't work on this—it will come.

3. Oneness, or unconditional love: This is the perhaps the most important aspect of enlightenment. Psychic powers, manifesting, and mystical visions are trivial, even useless, if love is not present. The flowering of the heart deepens enlightenment, bringing the experience of oneness with All That Is; or some days you suddenly feel causeless love for strangers, or feel like everything is inside of you or that you are indistinguishable from everything. You might talk directly with nature, bring rain, communicate with animals, or somehow know what someone needs. You tap into Universal Intelligence to know useful things in your areas of interest, whether it's science, car repair, or business. There is no longer any sense of separation between you and All That Is. You're aware that you are a distinct part of All That Is. It usually comes in peaks, but you are forever transformed unless you choose to "go back to sleep."

With some things in life, you might want someone to tell you what to expect, give you the benefit of their experience; but you are urged to go into this very personal spiritual adventure open to discover the unique gift The Divine has for you. You cannot fail at this, and perfection is not the goal of this ever-expanding universe, nor is it a qualification for enlightenment. There will be more on this topic as the book progresses and as you go through your experience.

Once you've begun the unfolding of enlightenment, it's like being on a plane from New York to California; you can't get off the plane, so there's no need to stress about whether you'll get there or not. You can't make the journey go faster by running up and down the aisles, so you might as well relax and enjoy the ride. Each stage has its own sweetness, so enjoy it. You will arrive at the scheduled time!

There are classic signs, but your enlightenment will be unique.

Powers and Mystical Phenomena

POWERS AND MYSTICAL phenomena are wonderful talents and useful gifts, but they are not synonymous with enlightenment. One who can perform impressive feats, give psychic information, heal or see guides or other dimensional beings, but still withholds love from family members or loved ones, or lives in scarcity, conflict and fearfulness, has still not yet experienced the flowering of enlightenment.

As your enlightenment unfolds, you may be expecting to see or hear certain things that you've heard or read about, such as visions, voices, entities, angels, masters or light phenomena. You might. You might not. If you'll release all your concepts of what a spiritual or religious experience should be, you'll appreciate and enjoy your own unique experience more. Comparing, and expecting someone else's experiences to happen to you is a setup for disappointment. No two people's enlightenment will be the same, or look the same, nor should it.

Some will see other dimensions and auras, and know spiritual entities, angels, guides, or even "see God." Others will never have any such experience. Personally, I don't experience manifestations of Spirit as separate from myself. They occur for me as my Large Self speaking. To separate them and label them as some "other" seems artificial. Why have a division between the spiritual and the material? Why separate the daily mundane life and the spiritual life? The more you can experience it fresh, the purer and more distortion-free it will be.

Consider that angels, guides, beings, and even visions of God are all *manifest forms*, while the purest essence of The Creator is *formless*, and pre-manifest. In the deepest oneness with The Presence, there is nothing but the silence of The Void. Enlightened singer/composer Miten says in his song, *Empty Heart*, "I tried to name the nameless. I tried hard to understand. When I closed my fist, well of course I missed. There was nothing in my hand. I've got this empty heart, that I can't explain. No longing for love, no sweet pain. No voice I hear in the still of night, just an empty heart, full of light." Find Deva Premal and Miten's music at www.devapremalmiten.com.

I encourage you to clean out all your old concepts of what you think spirituality is, and what you think God is. If no one had influenced you—if no one had written books about it—what would you experience? There is plenty of research showing that people experience God as their culture has trained them to. There is little variation within each culture's experience, but there is drastic variation between cultures. In mystical experiences, Christians see Jesus or Mary or angels. In the East no one ever sees them! They see Krishna or Ganesha, Mohammed or Buddha.

What if you gave up concepts such as angels, guides and other labels? What if you forget what books, your culture and other people said, and have a direct, personal experience of your Creator? You could have your first-ever pure, authentic spiritual experience. People are often so busy looking for something they read about, that they miss their own experience!

For many like myself, the deepest experiences are of pure feeling, or the silence, and if you're looking for something more visual or flashy, you can miss the deepest experiences of all. It will eventually become so intense that you cannot miss it, so don't worry. When the bliss body lights up, it feels ecstatic just to breathe. And then you'll get used to it.

One morning I woke up and felt physically and emotionally bad. So I relaxed into the feeling to experience it fully, so it could move up to a higher vibration. Within ten minutes not only did it move, but I was in such deep bliss that I laid there for another half hour just luxuriating in it. Those experiences are far more common for me than flashy phenomena, and I love them. I would not trade with anyone. They're mine. Have yours.

You will soon not only accept, but also love the reality you have! What every human being wants is to feel good and be happy, and once you have that, you won't care what form it takes.

Savor your unique experience and it will deepen and expand.

Design Your Own Enlightenment

ONE OF MY GREATEST fears about going to India was that I'd come out of it so blissed out that I would not be able to live in this world, relate to regular people, and deal with the practical day to day aspects of life. Then I learned we could design our enlightenment however we wanted. I had apprehensions about the program being extreme or cultish. Then I learned that there would be no dogma, nothing to believe in, no practices to do, no one to follow, and no rules binding me once I left there. That wasn't entirely the case, as there was a giving away of too much power to the gurus, but I took the part I wanted and left the rest. There is no dogma or rules in Divine Openings, only teachings that you might find helpful on your journey.

The last fear, the fear of losing my "separate self" or personality, I would have to deal with. On the one hand I knew that all our problems are self-created, and that it is that small separate self that causes all of them. But isn't it funny how we don't trust The Divine, our Large Self, the unlimited part of us, to know what's best for us? We trust our car to start, the sun to come up in the morning, and the airplane to stay aloft, but we don't trust God! It was weird, knowing that surrender to The Divine was the way to go, but not fully wanting to do it. That's how humanity has gotten in the state it's in, being separate from God and determined to do it "our way" even if it's the hard way.

I was so strongly called to go to India, to do an unknown process with people I didn't know, that I decided to just put one foot in front of the other. It was soothing news that we could design our own enlightenment, and that no two people's enlightenment would be alike. Some were asking for mystical experiences and cosmic consciousness. Some actually wanted to be erased, and that was an option if you asked for it; fine for them, but that wasn't for me. People who had been erased were sometimes barely functional in the world. That's OK for a monk, esoteric teacher or someone who wasn't interested in the material world, but I was clear that I wanted full engagement in the world. The enlightenment I designed and prayed to The Divine for was a practical one that would have me be effective in business, relationships, and all aspects of the material world.

If you can let go of any concepts about what enlightenment is you'll find that an authentic enlightenment unfolds for you. Most of the literary accounts and known examples are of spiritual teachers, but not everyone is meant to be a spiritual teacher. Enlightened people are now holding down high tech jobs, driving buses, filling prescriptions, and raising children. My dream is to see enlightened people in all walks of life and in all professions; it's not just for mystics, spiritual teachers, and healers, although that's the stereotype we expect. I see people suffering unnecessarily over their careers, struggling unsuccessfully to be healers or teachers when that is not their path.

We need enlightened people in all roles in life, from bakers baking with love, to maids cleaning with intention, to CEO's leading enlightened corporations. I fully plan to be out of a job when everyone is self-guided and awake. Maybe I'll be a joy-generating singer. So please don't succumb to the popular mania that you would be happier or more fulfilled in some other career that has more spiritual "significance." I had given up teaching, knowing full well that being an artist would be just as good. Then surprisingly, I was called from within to return to teaching. Folks, if you're called to teach or heal, you will not be able to stop yourself! I can attest to this. If that doesn't flow for you, pay close attention to what does flow, and be happy. You make a difference for others in any career.

Just as in my concept of God, in my enlightenment I wanted to include lots of humor and fun, playfulness and spontaneity. A real cowgirl is not the least bit interested in qualities like saintliness and piety. I wanted only enough gravity to be credible and taken seriously; my gift is more to lighten people up than to be the serious, heavy type—how boring! Each of us is a broadcast tower in our daily lives. We're always beaming something out there whether we're doing business consulting, serving food, or repairing someone's car. Enlightenment makes you a beacon no matter what you're doing. There is no profession unworthy of an enlightened person, or lesser than any other profession. If you enjoy it and are good at it, it's valuable. I'd like to see farming become an enlightened profession, with farmers who are one with the land, plants, animals, and ecosystem, and produce vibrant, healthy food, and a clean environment. One Divine Openings Giver who runs a farm in northern California can direct the cattle with her mind.

So how might your enlightenment be? What would you like to include in it, and what would you like to leave out? Spend a few moments wondering. Of course you will discover new parts of yourself that you cannot now imagine once it begins to unfold, and you can keep revising it forever. But have a little fun now daydreaming about it. You are a powerful creator, even a miracle worker, in your fully enlightened state. What might you do with that?

ACTIVITY: Write in your journal now. Imagine the most ideal world, and your most wonderful place in it, just for fun. Be open to unknown possibilities. Drop it completely and let go before you do the next Divine Opening. Take nothing with you.

Divine Opening

GAZE FOR TWO minutes, then close your eyes, lie down, and let go.

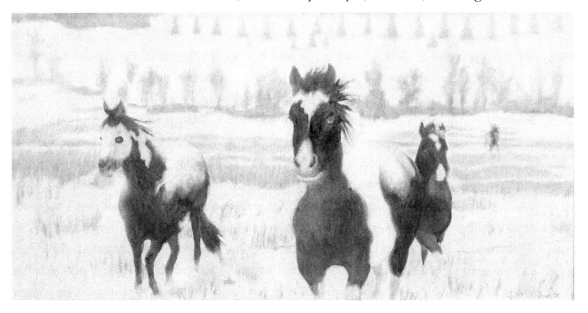

Figure 6—Ghost Horses, a painting by Lola Jones.

The art is shown in color in the Art Gallery at www.DivineOpenings.com.

8 ½ x 11" printable files or large archival prints can be purchased on the site as well.

Between Worlds

WE STRADDLE TWO dimensions—the older dimension in which we have to massage our thoughts and feelings to get them up or to keep them at a high altitude—and the next dimension of life that is opening up, in which our enlightened minds produce thoughts and feelings of a very high altitude more of the time. In the old world we had to work hard to force enlightened thought because our brains were not wired to sustain it. Now Divine Openings literally plugs us into our Larger Intelligence, activates our higher capacities, and upgrades our systems so that we can run "enlightenment software." When we're no longer slaves to our thoughts and feelings, nor unduly identified with them, it's easier to stay up. We have still have Free Will choices, though.

Enlightened beings still experience contrasts of wanted and unwanted experiences, but tend to use the unwanted experiences as fuel to propel them with more velocity toward their desired choices. We bounce off of the unwanted things like we bounce a cue ball off the side of a pool table to sink the bank shot. During this awakening process most people find that they wobble until they stabilize. One day you may feel peace and oneness, and the next day you may experience extreme separation as old vibrations activate and move up. One day you may be blissed out, the next you may be depressed. There is really nothing for you to do except "experience your experience." It's all temporary and moves quickly. The day you fear no feeling you are free.

This book gives you the conscious mind piece and the Grace piece. You get tools you can use immediately to make the best of your Free Will choices, while the Divine Openings work on you and for you in ways that you could not do for yourself. I've taken you deeper into the Grace part, that gift that you cannot earn by your own efforts.

The next chapter deals with the conscious mind piece, and introduces you to your "Instrument Panel," navigating, and "keeping your altitude up." The conscious mind pieces are not from my twenty-one days of silence. It sythesized over several decades, from my dreams, my corporate courses, some from the work of Esther and Jerry Hicks and others, but the bulk of it was more recently inspired from within. The Large Self/small self concept, I developed eighteen years ago for the corporate world. Now I find clients move much more rapidly when we retrain the conscious-mind in addition to evoking Divine Grace. It helps the mind understand where the Large Self is leading, and reduces mind interference.

How To Navigate

THE NEXT SECTION gives the fundamentals of steering your life and manifesting your desires. If you have difficulty letting in the things you want in life, consider this: an enlightened person who is fulfilled and prosperous, and whose own needs are met, has more power and ability to make a difference in the world. Struggling to pay your bills and buy gas puts you in survival mode, and being in a low vibration doesn't help you be a light in the world.

Decades ago, for many years, I had a recurring dream in which I had a "control panel" that I used to guide my spaceship. Upon waking, it dissolved from my hands, even as I grasped desperately for it, and it felt awful. In later years, thank God, I found my long-lost control panel and gained constant access to it. I'm about to re-introduce you to your long-lost control panel.

On my flight to and from India, a TV screen in front of each seat showed our aircraft on a map of the world, alternating with a screen with flight statistics, so I always knew where we were, how far away we were from the destination, the velocity, altitude, and direction of the flight.

With the control panel back in my hands, life has become like that. It is no longer a blind flight, landing in some unpleasant place, wondering how I got there. Now I always know how I got there. Soon it will be quite clear to you too.

Once you rediscover your marvelous control panel or "Instrument Panel," you will never again be confused, lost, or off-course for long. You will move surely toward the rendezvous point you desire, and you will know in plenty of time if you need to change your route or altitude to avoid a collision or make your desired landing. You will never again be mystified by why anything happened, because you will see exactly how you navigated there, even if it was unintentional or unconscious. You'll know exactly where you are headed, how fast you are going to get there, and how it will feel once you get there. The past will make sense, and you'll use it for the future.

Knowing where my Instrument Panel is, and checking it constantly, I know exactly what I'm creating and where I am headed in any given moment. If I feel bad, I know I'm pointing the nose of the plane at the ground, and where I'm headed will also feel bad. If I feel good, I know I'm pointing the nose of the plane upward. I'm headed where I want to go, and it will feel good.

Keep the nose of the plane tipped up.

Your Instrument Panel

FOR YEARS WE were told that our thoughts create our reality—that we get what we think about. No wonder we got so frustrated when it didn't always work. We didn't have our Instrument Panel.

Read this section slowly. Even if you have read fifty books on Law of Attraction and think you already know this, there's more here.

Conscious and unconscious thoughts vibrate. Vibration broadcasts out from you like a radio tower. It attracts similar vibrations to you—people, places, and things that match your vibration. If you're broadcasting sadness, then more sad experiences, people, places, things are attracted to you. If you're *authentically* broadcasting happiness, then more happy experiences, people, places and things are attracted to you.

Your Creator gave you feelings to help you know the vibrations you are broadcasting. Those feelings tell you how closely you are in alignment with your Large Self, or God Self, and so are miraculous predictors of the reality you're creating next. If you are feeling the higher emotions about your desired destination, feeling relaxed and allowing yourself to be guided and carried along by life, you are in alignment with your Large Self, the larger-perspective you, on that subject. Being your Large Self feels better, and gets you where you want to go faster.

Being your small self and feeling the lower emotions isn't *wrong*, it just isn't as powerful. Your Large Self is always at a high altitude, which means your Large Self always feels good, so if you feel good you are in alignment with your Large Self. If you are feeling bad, you are simply out of alignment with your Large Self. That is *supposed to feel bad!* Soon you will always know why your actions and plans are working or not working. You will always know where you are and which way is "up." With full use of your Instrument Panel, you'll always know whether you are in alignment with your Large Self—and if you're not, how to get back there.

Soon you'll know without a doubt whether you are headed toward your goal or away from it. Once you get re-calibrated to your Instrument Panel, you will never be "lost" again. Like the flight screen on my transatlantic voyage, it takes the mystery out of where you are, and how far you have yet to go. When you know where you are, it's easier to navigate to where you want to go in life.

Emotions are a continuum, from very low vibrational feelings like grief, fear, sadness and despair all the way up to joy, love, appreciation, even ecstasy. Rather than make a detailed list of the progression from bottom to top, let's start out with the general idea—the goal is to move up the Instrument Panel and feel better—even a little better helps.

If you're in fear, despair, anger, frustration or any lower emotion, we'll call that a "low altitude." You want to gain altitude slowly and steadily, rising up the Instrument Panel, feeling a little better at each level. Just go for a slightly better feeling, a slightly higher altitude. Stabilize there, and then move on up. Momentum becomes your friend once you get an upward trend going.

Your Instrument Panel because tells you where you are *on a given subject*. Your Large Self vibrates up at the top of the Instrument Panel all the time, so "up" is toward your Large Self. At the top of the scale is POWER. When you're up there you have access to all of your power and all of the power of your Large Self. That's a lot of power. Aim up there where your Large Self is—but again, it's *easier to do it incrementally*, one step at a time, and it's longer lasting.

You're at different levels on the Instrument Panel on different topics. For example: you might be at a high altitude about money and friends, and at a lower altitude about romantic relationship. Therefore your financial and social life is great but your romantic life is not so fulfilling.

The Instrument Panel translates your feelings to altitude readings. It helps you remember what you knew when you were little. You knew how to read your feelings from your own Instrument Panel and naturally find your way up through the feelings, and to rise in altitude. A child, if allowed to do what it wants, naturally knows how to move up in altitude. But most people lose touch with their own Instrument Panel over time from listening to other people instead of trusting their own readings.

The important thing is to feel what is "up" or "down" for *you* rather than following my description of the feelings to the letter. Most people find the Instrument Panel pretty accurate, but some of you place some emotions in slightly different spots, and that's OK. Words are not precise. Feelings are very accurate predictors.

Whatever feels better to you is "up."

You don't even have to name the emotion -- just feel it and note whether it feels good or bad to you, and note which way is up. Naming the emotion is most useful is when you suddenly realize that frustration, while it still feels bad, is not that low! You might notice that you've moved up from an unworthy feeling to frustration, and that actually calls for a celebration.

The biggest choice, in any given moment, is whether to let the Large Self or the small self fly the plane. There is no bad place to be on the Instrument Panel or as a human being. It is all valuable information. You are where you are and The Presence never judges you. Once you know how to navigate, you can get anywhere you want to go from anywhere you are.

If you're in Los Angeles and you'd rather live in New York, get a map, get in your car and point it toward New York. You know it's a long journey, but you know you'll get there. Your life will be more like that now. You can navigate. You can predict how long it will be till something you want arrives by how you feel about it, and which way you're pointed. If you feel ecstatic about it, you know you'll be there soon. If you feel doubtful about it, you're not quite pointed at it. If you're depressed about it, you're headed away from it.

You'll feel negative things coming from miles away, and have plenty of time to change your attitude, altitude, and alter your course to avoid colliding with those negative events. When you feel bad, you'll be able to say, "Hmmm, I know this is not leading somewhere I want to go, so how do I lift my altitude and adjust my course?"

Summary: there are no "bad" emotions. They're all indicators of alignment or misalignment with your Large Self as regards your desire. Emotions are valuable information to tell you where you're pointed. There's much more, and we'll take it one step at a time.

Get Yourself To The Party

WHEN YOU DESIRE something, your Large Self instantly tunes into your vibration, and creates it in the non-physical. Snap! Done! Your Large Self starts that particular party for you right then and there. Ninety-nine percent of your desire is manifested and waiting for you—at the party. Where are you? Your job is only this: to get where you Large Self is on that subject, high on the Instrument Panel—and get yourself to the party. You're the guest of honor, the party is poised, ninety-nine percent complete, ready to begin. The band is set up, the food is on the table, the guests are all standing there, waiting for you, the guest of honor. But this party can't start without *you,* because it's *your party.* Are you the missing element at your own party? Do you think about the parties you didn't get to in the past, how there probably won't be any party, or no one will come, or something will go wrong—and hold yourself back from your own party?

Or do you let go of all those contradictory vibrations, ignore your mind's doubts, and focus with all your heart on the party? Talk about the party, and ways to get there. Talk about what you want rather than what you fear, and you'll get to the party *faster!* That last puzzle piece that completes the party is you. I want to make a T-shirt that says, "I *AM* the party!"

I'm not saying never talk to anyone about your challenges, but do it sparingly, because *as you speak, you create.* Commiseration is co-misery, and plummets your altitude. If you must, speak your challenge quickly, and then shift your words to what you want, solutions, and possibilities. I rarely ever speak of problems to friends. Why? Direct-to-The-Presence is the most powerful place to go with questions or challenges. Friendship is not about emotional support or problem-solving for me at all anymore. When I'm with friends and loved ones, the focus is on living, loving, and fun.

Get to the party!

Your Instrument Panel.

Ecstasy   **YOU FEEL POWERFUL UP HERE.**

Joy, Bliss   Your Large Self vibrates up here all the time.

Direct Knowing, Empowerment   This energy is light, fast, flowing, un-resisted.

Freedom   Each step up feels more powerful.

Love, Appreciation

Passion, Eagerness, Enthusiasm

Happiness, Positive Expectation   **More Expansive Energy**

Belief   The party's up here!

Optimism, Confidence, I Can Do It

Hopefulness, Seeing Possibilities, Curiosity

Self Esteem, Interest, Courage

Contentment, Relaxation, Emptiness

Acceptance, Boredom, I Don't Care ------- The resting zone, not exciting, but useful.

Pessimism, I Give Up

------------------ THE TIPPING POINT--------------------

Frustration, Aggravation, Impatience

Overwhelm, Stressed, Overwork   Much of society lives here and thinks it's normal.

Disappointment

Doubt, Confusion, Uncertainty

Worry, Negative expectation

Discouragement, I Cannot Do It, Fatigue

Anger --- A bridge to get your power/energy back.

Revenge

Hatred, Rage   **More Contracted Energy**

Jealousy, Desire That Feels Bad, Lack   Get up there to the party!

Guilt, Blame, Projecting Negativity On Others

Fear   **YOU FEEL POWERLESS DOWN HERE.**

Sadness   The energy is slow, heavy, dense, resistant.

Grief, Depression   It's hard to hear your Large Self down here.

Shame, Unworthiness, Despair, Apathy

Every emotion on the Instrument Panel is Divine Energy at varying frequencies.
All emotions are valuable information. Appreciate them all!

Much appreciation and love to Esther and Jerry Hicks, David R. Hawkins, and others whose emotional/consciousness scales helped me rediscover my long lost "control panel."

Everything is Divine energy, but the vibratory rate of the emotions at the bottom of the Instrument Panel is lower, relative to the un-resisted, higher, faster vibrations at the top. As you move up the Altimeter, vibration is faster, less dense. There's light, power, velocity, and vitality. As you move down, it's more sluggish and dense. There's less light, power, velocity and vitality.

It's supposed to feel bad at the bottom of the Instrument Panel—that tells you you've gotten out of alignment with your Large Self. It feels good to be at the top of the Instrument Panel because you're in alignment and agreement with your true, powerful Large Self. You obviously cannot get completely separated from your Large Self—that's impossible, you're part of it—but at the bottom you're relatively off your Large Self's frequency and at the top you're right on it.

Look at the Instrument Panel and *feel* in your body the levels of energy as they increase from the bottom upward. When you stop resisting feeling, that energy rises in frequency, and gets more organized and Intelligent. Then you feel better. Then things go better. Resistance is simply contracted, pinched off energy, as opposed to expansive, flowing, high vibrational energy.

The small self is by nature fearful, doubtful, and resistant, and has no interest in giving up control and going with the flow, but your *intention* to feel good and put the Large Self in the driver's seat prevails over time. Be soft and compassionate with your small self, which is doing the best it can with its limited consciousness. It is fear-based, and so might resist anything unknown, just because it's new, even if the new is clearly better.

From your Large Self perspective, make the decision to soothe the small self and have it take a back seat. *Choose and decide* to let your Large Self fly the plane and orchestrate it all. It has a larger perspective and unlimited resources. It IS your Source.

Let your Large Self fly the plane.

ACTIVITY: Get up and act out the Instrument Panel on the previous page from bottom to top, using your body. This is especially useful if you are having difficulty feeling. Physical movement un-sticks you quickly, by taking you from dry concept to active experience. *Do* the activities if you want the maximum effects. Make it silly and fun and uninhibited. Which ones have slower or faster energy? Write in your journal how it felt and anything you noticed.

Did you get up and move, or did you resist? Go back if you didn't do the activity. Most people have gotten so used to negative emotion that they think it's normal, and just sit in it. No wonder they get nasty surprises! First priority: get back in touch with your feelings and get your Altimeter calibrated again. Notice during your day, "I feel this, I feel that." "This is what I feel." No faking. You are where you are. Don't make it bad and don't try to change it; let it be what it is.

It's all just information. Wherever you are is OK, because from this day forward, by looking at your Instrument Panel, you will know which way is up. When you're caught up in stories about how you got there, whose fault it is, and how powerless you are to change it, do those thoughts make you feel better, or worse? The game is to soothe yourself and tell yourself a better "story," one that leads to even a slight rise in altitude, a few steps up the Instrument Panel. Easy does it. One step at a time is all it takes.

"Truth" is not the issue here. Where you are is "true" only because you created it, or you bought into a reality someone else created. You made it true. It's temporarily true till you create something else! You can now create something else you like and make that "true." Changing your story about it helps you feel more powerful, and feeling powerful creates powerful realities.

Check your Instrument Panel to see where you are, what your altitude is, which way you're headed, and how you might need to adjust to end up where you want to go. The altitude on your airplane's Instrument Panel is neither wrong nor right; it's simply information. If you don't like what you see, make adjustments. You have Free Will. Use it wisely.

Using your Instrument Panel, you can get anywhere. If you don't use it, you often end up in unexpected places, experiencing things you don't want, and wondering why. But the good news is, if you point at San Francisco and keep the nose tipped up, not down, you *will arrive there*.

Summary: Unwanted or "negative" emotions are useful data. They tell you where you are. You're supposed to feel bad when the nose of your plane is tipped even slightly downward, so you're alerted to the long-term consequences. A slight tipping up of the nose of your plane is huge. It changes the outcome of your entire journey, and eventually, your life.

It's not important to get to the highest altitude right away—just get the nose tipped up a bit. Get headed in the general direction you want to go. Just go for a little feeling of relief, or improvement in how you feel. You must value small gains. Small gains mean everything in the long run.

Point your nose upward and relax.

One day I was happily writing, but as time to teach a class approached the nose tipped down as I thought about having to stop writing. I noticed the drop and adjusted my focus to how much fun it would be to start writing again after the class. I reminded myself how much fun classes are. Downward spirals start in such innocent ways, but that's all it takes to tip the nose back up.

Once you know how to use the readings your built-in Instrument Panel gives you, every moment of every day, you'll feel things coming to you from miles away, and you'll have plenty of time to adjust your trajectory in time to either merge with a desired target or avoid an unwanted collision. You will have full awareness of what you're creating long before the creation is complete, simply by noticing how you feel **about that subject,** instead of realizing after the creation is complete that your altitude **on that subject** had been low. You'll also get the bliss before the wanted thing arrives, so you won't even be surprised when fabulous things show up.

If you are feeling good about a subject, and your nose is pointed up, you're gonna like the manifestation that you're cooking up. If you're feeling bad about a subject, and your nose is pointed down, you're probably not gonna like the manifestation you're lining up. How much better is it to be able to feel and forecast your results in advance? As you get more attuned to feeling, you'll have plenty of time to get in alignment with your Large Self and so achieve the outcome you want.

If you're in depression or frustration or at any lower altitude, now you know that to get back to being your Large Self you need to point the nose up and move up the Instrument Panel.

The game is to move up the scale and feel a little better. We've been told for so long that feeling bad is just the human condition; we believed we were supposed to gut it up and tolerate a lot of feeling bad. So we allowed ourselves to stay at low altitudes, not realizing how damaging that is over time. Even when something bad happens, feeling bad won't get you anything, even if everyone agrees how wronged you were. That victim feeling attracts more victimization. It's not worth the measly reward of being right. Take the controls, tip the nose up, and you change your course now. Changing how you feel now changes your tomorrow. Notice where you are, and then "intend" to climb.

Decades ago, in that recurring dream where I had my "control panel" in my hands, I felt powerful. Upon awaking, I'd panic as it slipped out of my fingers and faded. Now I often have abstract dreams of esoteric knowledge that eludes me as I wake. It's fun to wonder what new revelations will come out of those dreams in time. Notice that I'm not lamenting the inability to know right now. Now I know it does translate eventually. I'm playfully curious, and savoring the waiting.

Make a lifelong decision that feeling better
is the most important thing in the world.

Step By Step

IF YOU'RE LOW on the Instrument Panel on a particular subject, your job is not to get to ecstasy about it today. That's too hard. Your job is to feel just a little bit better today and a little bit better tomorrow. You can do that. Some people get frustrated and quit when they can't get to joy today, or to skinny today, or to debt-free today. But think about it: would you expect a baby to learn to walk in one day or even one week? Would you expect to train for a marathon in one month after being out of shape for five years? NO! *Your success depends on being happy with small steps.* Those small steps will take you there, and when you get there you'll be stable and you'll stay up there.

When you move "up" there's a slight feeling of relief, of gaining energy.

If you are feeling just a tiny bit better about money today, more money is coming in the days and weeks to follow. If you are feeling just a little bit better about your body today, a better body is coming. If you get discouraged, you split and contradict your energy, and your result is delayed because materialization follows vibration. Sweating it adds more negativity that contradicts your pure desire! Relax. Tip the nose up. Get yourself to the party.

Make the most of the best, and the least of the worst.

Here's how a step-by-step altitude-raising conversation with yourself might sound. Note where she is on the Altimeter **(in bold)** and how she moves up slowly and stabilizes at each point:

"I just feel **worthless.** If I were worth anything, Bill would love me. I can't muster any energy to change my life. Wow, I'm low on the Instrument Panel. Now I know where I am, and I want to tip the nose up. Knowing where I am gives me direction. OK, where I am is where I am, so I'll be with this, and now I know what I want—to feel better about myself!"

"I'm **sad and depressed** because Bill doesn't seem to love me. Even if it's true, he's just one person, although he seems like the only one for me. Being sad feels bad, but what's worse is, I am out of sync with my Large Self down here. I'm not at the party. But... I am where I am!"

"I'm **angry** about this powerlessness! I want my power back! What is he, stupid? Can't he see? Oh, that's good. I'm breathing and my energy is returning. Whew, I think I'll take a walk and feel this anger. I'll be with it and not talk to him or anyone about it. I hate this! No more!"

Next day: "I'm **discouraged,** but that's up from anger. Yes! Hmm, well at least I know where I am—closer to the party! I'll take a break from relationships until I get clearer. I give up; it's too discouraging to keep trying because my old story about relationships is creating the same old outcome. I'm practicing a new way to be. Onward to the party!"

"I could try soothing myself before I talk to him, then I'll come from a place that's easier to hear. If I am easy on myself, that softening moves me up just a bit. I can do that. Ahhh."

"That feels better—not great, but better. Better is all I need for this moment."

"I am **confused** that I don't know what to do about this complicated situation. It's too **overwhelming** to try to talk to him just yet. We've said too many words already."

"It's **frustrating** when I've tried so many things so many times. Ahh, I've been trying to manipulate him into loving me! I hate feeling frustrated, but I will be with it!"

"Maybe I can just **accept** who and how he is, let go, and let God handle it. I'm **bored** with the whole thing—forget about him for a while. I'm going dancing."

Next week: "Ah, letting go works. This feels **hopeful** at least. I don't have to figure it out, but I can daydream about the **possibilities.** If it's not him, then there's someone better for me, who adores me. I feel relief right now. I think I'll go do something productive while my Large Self handles it. I'll get a feeling if there's any action for me to take."

When you feel even slight relief, claim a victory. If you were out of shape and started training for a marathon, you would have to be happy with small daily improvements, or you would never make it. This is the same. For now, practice just to gain confidence that you can move even slightly.

Don't focus on changing your outer world or your results for now. That's too large a step. Just feel a tiny bit better each day and let Grace do ninety percent of it. Your ten percent is to use your Free Will to point the nose up. Fretting only points the nose down. Focus on being happy and letting go. Outer changes come naturally as you change inside. They have to—it is a Law of the Universe.

Raise your altitude *just because it feels better,* rather than because you want the guy, the girl, the job, the house, or the money. Do it for you. Do it because you've decided feeling as good as you can in this moment is vital. Your life will always be *this moment,* and if you are a little bit happier in this moment, and this moment, and this moment, you change the trajectory of your life. Maybe you can't manage outer circumstances, but you can *choose* how to *focus* in this moment.

Stop focusing on outer results. Focus on letting go and feeling better.

There is no top limit to how far up you can go, so it isn't just about getting out of pain and struggle. Getting out of pain and struggle is just step one. You can create ever-increasing joy. When you were young—you felt the truth of the Altimeter. You knew how to move up it naturally. I am here to remind you of what you knew, before you were convinced to ignore your own inner guidance. Master this and be your Large Self playing in material reality, consciously and joyfully— full out.

Soothe yourself. Today's feelings create tomorrow's reality.

ACTIVITY: Each night at bedtime, write in your journal any positive steps you made. Briefly give your cares, worries, and missteps to The Presence. Let them go and don't retell the stories. Shift to Large Self perspective. Small steps are what most big successes are made of. *Don't listen to everything your mind says.* Pivot to encouraging thoughts and feelings. Write a story that moves you up in altitude small-step-by-small-step. Don't get too hung up on "reality." You created it! There is no obligation to stick to the truth or be "accurate." *You* created *it.*

For more practical processes, visit www.DivineOpenings.com/spiritual-enlightenment-processes.

The Power Is Not "Out There"

PEOPLE TOO OFTEN want to fix what's making them feel bad by changing something or someone "out there." They try to make someone change their behavior, talk it out, manipulate the circumstances, change jobs, make the world change—so they can be happy. But if the world has to change before you can be happy, you're in big, big trouble! There are too many people and too many things that would have to change, and have you ever managed to change even *one* person? Does your government have to change before you can be happy? Does your body have to change first? Does your income have to change first? Good luck!

Your world shifts when you shift. It's an inside job. Throwing action at it and trying to control people and circumstances won't change it. Change your altitude first. Hold off on actions and big decisions until you are happy and clear. If you act when your altitude is low, you'll work too hard or create things you don't want. Create in the non-physical, with intention and vibration first. Then take action as guided. Then your actions will be exponentially more effective.

You can cut your action to a fraction.

Just Because You Can't See It Yet

IT'S A GREAT cosmic joke that what is most real is invisible and non-physical. You can't always see, touch, hear, feel, or smell it. Love, energy, life force, compassion, magnetism, gravity, hope, and the intention and energy that always precedes physical materialization are invisible, but very powerfully real. The physical "reality" we can see and touch is much less real and lasting—it's fleeting and impermanent. As physicists know, things that seem to be solid and heavy really are not—they're mostly space. Your physical senses are now evolving to sense a broader spectrum of reality. You'll begin to see, hear, know, and feel more things that aren't physical. You'll be able to sense what's coming while it's still just a non-physical intention. The more sensitive you become to non-physical pre-manifest energy, the more you can tangibly feel things long before they pop into the physical. Now the non-physical world is much more real to me than the physical world.

You and a "realist" friend are standing outside looking at the thirsty trees and grass, and you really want some rain. You're surfing on a wave of happy anticipation of rain. A great storm just swells out of nowhere, fifty miles away, and you feel it coming. The realist says, "There's no rain in the forecast, I see no rain, and no rain's coming. We're in a drought." So what's the reality?

The money, love, or experience you want is there, even if you can't see it. Get on and ride the wave of its coming. You can enjoy it now. It's real. You created it.

What's most real is often invisible.

Sometimes I like to drive to the mountains. Three quarters of the way there, the flat road stretches out for fifty miles ahead without a curve in it. It looks nothing like the vacation we're aiming for. But of course we don't turn around just because we don't see a single shred of evidence with our eyes. The road signs say we're pointed in the right direction. We find ways to enjoy the drive—music, laughing, anticipating, stopping to take photographs or leisurely walks.

We're almost there before we spot even a few small foothills. Compared to my vision of snow-capped mountains it's not very exciting—pretty un-spectacular. We keep driving. It's the very last fraction of the drive before we actually see mountains. Wow, there they are, rising ten thousand feet or more. The air gets chilly and crisp; the scent of pine fills the air, and a cold, crystal clear stream winds alongside the highway. We see a lovely mountain cottage to stay in. It's been worth the drive.

Your journey can be like that. No evidence, no evidence, no evidence . . . then, BOOM! Big evidence. It snowballs, but you don't see it snowballing until the snowball rolls up to you.

The party is waiting for you. Just hang in there, keep going, and enjoy getting there. If you feel yourself flagging, losing hope, doubting, talk to yourself like you'd talk to any friend who was losing their direction: "The party's starting, but they're waiting for me! I don't have to do everything; the Divine does the heavy lifting. As long as I don't turn back, I'll get there. All I have to do is keep vibrating high, point in that general direction, keep rolling, and I will arrive."

Take score only when the score is in your favor.

Divine Opening

LOLA INVOKES a powerful Divine Mother vibration here.
You can enjoy as many of this Divine Mother Hug type of Divine Opening as you like, as often as you like, because they do not accelerate your energy and do not require assimilation time. They are soothing, calming, and grounding. Gaze, then close your eyes and relax.

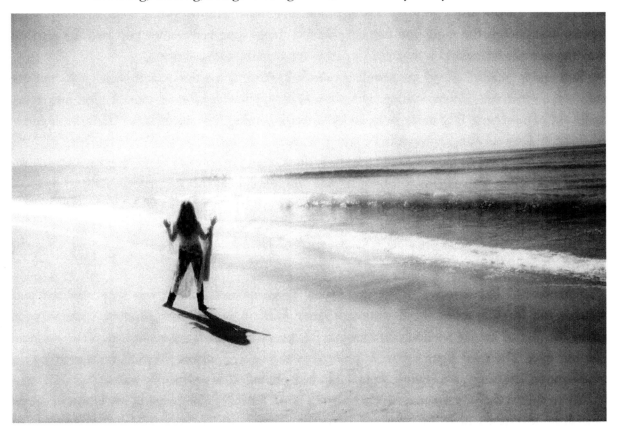

Figure 7—Lola Jones by the sea. A photograph by Carola Gracen.

All art is shown in color in the Art Gallery at www.DivineOpenings.com, but the black and white works the same. 8 ½ x 11" printable files or large archival prints can be purchased on the site.

Grace Supersedes Law of Attraction

THE BEST NEWS OF ALL is that Grace supersedes Law of Attraction, so you get free boosts to get you going, rather than having to ratchet your vibration up by working on it. Divine Openings is not a "do it all yourself" program like Law of Attraction, although we observe and use the Law of Attraction. With Divine Openings, the Divine does the heavy lifting. Grace does ninety percent. Your job, your ten percent is to train yourself to use your Free Will effectively to manage your vibration, because Law of Attraction attracts feelings, people, things, and experiences to match what you are already vibrating. If you're feeling bliss, Law of Attraction brings you more blissful feelings, people, things, and events. The Instrument Panel helps you pinpoint where you are on a particular subject, understand what you're attracting, and shift your vibration.

Like the laws of physics, Law of Attraction isn't personal. If Hitler and Gandhi both stood on a cliff and leaned forward, they would both fall and hit the ground. Gravity isn't personal, nor does it judge good or bad. Law of Attraction will help you stay high if you are high, but it will also contribute to keeping you at a low point if you are low. It has a "sticky" effect that pulls you back to the altitude that was your set point.

Like attracts like.

Law of Attraction and the Instrument Panel are not about how good or bad you're being—they're about your alignment with your Large Self. You're not "bad" for being out of alignment with your Large Self—it just doesn't feel good, and it leads to things you don't want. Give yourself compassion for where you are. Soften up on yourself and you instantly move up the Altimeter. Say to yourself, "I'm glad it doesn't feel good to be out of alignment with my Large Self!" You'll get an instant elevation. Appreciate that elevation and you get another one.

You're not good "because" you're at a high altitude—but when you're up there in alignment with your Large Self, you're headed someplace that you'll like. You're not bad at a low altitude—you're just pointed at destinations you won't like.

From depression, fear, sadness or despair, your inborn instincts know (or used to know) that anger is a powerful move upward. You were born with an instinct to get angry to get your power back when you get scared, sad, or depressed. As a child you knew anger felt better, more powerful than despair. But what were we told as children when we got angry? "You're being bad!" "Be nice." "You're going to get a spanking!" We'd get angry, get bad reactions from people, and then stuff it and go back down to depression; then our natural instincts to get angry would kick back in and we'd get angry, then someone would say we shouldn't do that. We'd ping-pong: anger, depression, anger, depression—or anger, fear, anger, fear—so we'd spin in circles and never make it all the way up the Altimeter. Some of us messed up our Instrument Panel and got it turned upside down.

Let yourself use the bridge of anger, and you can ease up to frustration. From there you can rise to hope, and so on, until you're flying higher, up there as your Large Self. It is best to keep anger, revenge and blame conversations internal. If you talk to your friends they'll just take your side and support your "story," and that won't help. Take it to The Presence. Your anger will soon pass, leaving you with more productive feelings. When we speak angry feelings to the other person it just escalates, and dumps our negativity on them. If they don't know how to raise their altitude they may have a hard time letting it go later, even though you've moved up the scale and now feel great. Raise your altitude first, and then speak to them from your Large Self; if you have something tough to say you'll say it more effectively, more lovingly. Your Large Self can say tough things with compassion and people might even thank you later!

Lower emotion is usually for internal use only.

People want us to do what feels good to them, not what feels good to us, and we get in a bind if we care more about what they think than what we know. As a result, in childhood many of us got our Instrument Panel so out of whack we couldn't read it anymore. "I love this, but mom says it's bad," or "This feels bad to me but my teacher says it's good." Up was down and down was up— which way do I go to feel better?

Some of us unplugged our Instrument Panel, numbed out, or ignored its signals, put a big fake smile on our face, and marched on, continually surprised at the things that happened to us that didn't make any sense because we didn't feel them coming. We had no clue how we got there since we didn't have any Instrument Panel readings.

Because of the sticky effect, the mind rejects affirmations that are too far from what you now believe; the leap from depression to joy is too big to sustain it. If your body or feelings say, "You're lying," you're trying to make too big a jump. Go for a more modest jump you can "buy." Talking cheery talk that you don't feel doesn't raise your altitude; it just fools you into thinking you're tipping the nose up when you're not, and the ground is still rising to meet you. Take it step by step. When you go slower and stabilize at each new higher altitude, Law of Attraction supports you, you don't fall back, and you eventually stick at the new higher set point.

While I didn't fully understand Law of Attraction at the time, I now realize how it factored into the dilemma with the attorney. The sticky effect of my old vibration made it difficult to leap up to making that much money at once from one project. On the subject of money I had a mixed vibration at that time: victim mixed with hopefulness. I had just finished some work where I'd felt disempowered. Now I remember feeling nervous when the attorney first gave me the work. My head was saying, "Oh, yeah, I'm confident. I have the job—this is good, ignore those fears." while my gut was vibrating, "Something's not right here," but I didn't know what it all meant. Today, I would never ignore a feeling and say, "Feel the fear and do it anyway." I would either raise the vibration first before taking it on, or not do it. Your real power comes when you begin to feel what you're attracting *while you're attracting it,* and so have time to raise your altitude in time to change it.

Practice until you can keep your focus on something you want without sticky contradictory thoughts pulling you back. When you can enjoy that feeling for just a few minutes without contradicting it you are on the way to mastering attraction.

You're never standing still—you're either very subtly spiraling upward or downward at any given moment, since Law of Attraction's sticky effect is compounding *whatever* you're vibrating.

Blind Spots

WHILE GRACE DOES supersede Law of Attraction and gives you unearned boosts in altitude, you can be sure Law of Attraction isn't ever cheating you. We're never victims. Life does make sense. Even if I don't know *how* I created something, as soon as I can muster it, I *claim* I created it, because saying I didn't create it makes me a victim. I don't *blame* myself for creating it, either; that's *self-victimization*. I take responsibility, not blame, and that restores my power instantly. I can use that power to move forward and create something I like better.

When your vibration on a subject is up, but you still haven't received what you want, it's right there for you. You're either taking score too soon (and vibrating lack) or you're broadcasting energy that you don't know you're broadcasting. I call that a blind spot. You've been practicing some vibrational habits for so long you don't know you're doing it. You've stopped noticing that some things feel bad—or you unplugged your Instrument Panel. You've become numb to certain things or have come to accept that they are "normal." Feeling bad is *not normal*. Get help if you suspect you have blind spots. See www.DivineOpenings.com for session information.

We've picked up beliefs and vibrations we didn't know we picked up. We didn't mean to. Whole cultures and families vibrate things unconsciously, like prosperity or poverty, peace or violence, worthiness or unworthiness. If you don't choose awakening, the world pulls you in un-chosen directions, and consensus reality makes those blind spots seem normal. When everyone's doing it, it's harder to see it. Blind spots are invisible. It only occurred to me after Divine Openings just how extremely warlike as a collective America is. Some countries don't fight; it's just not in their collective consciousness. Some countries have a victim vibration, and get abused by other countries, or even by their own people or leaders.

Divine Openings gradually opens your eyes to things you couldn't see before.

Unconscious broadcasts (blind spots) attract, too.

As doves are thrown aloft into the air during celebrations—Grace lifts you aloft, and does ninety percent of it for you on the non-physical level. You still have to flap your wings here and there, and point your beak where you want to go. Do your ten percent: make conscious choices, use your Free Will wisely, keep the nose tipped up, and take the action you're guided to take. As you practice Divine Openings you'll be able to let in more Grace— the gift that cannot be "earned" by one's own efforts. Grace has been raining on you all along, but if you can't let it in you can feel like you're drowning even in a rainstorm. As Divine Openings expands your pipes you can let in more Grace and ease.

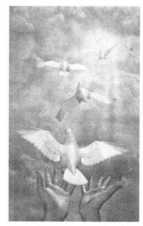

A Steady Climb For Lasting Results

GRACE GIVES YOU those free boosts of peace or bliss, and then you must use your Free Will choices to stay up there. After each burst of bliss, at first Law of Attraction might nudge you back down a bit, toward your old, established set point. Your set point is sticky, so it tends to pull you back down a bit after big gains in altitude. Incremental rises are easier to sustain. That's all you can do sometimes, and it's enough to matter. If you judge it "not enough," that sends you sliding further down in altitude. Appreciate small gains. Appreciation always gets you extra altitude.

Law of Attraction is on your side once you've stabilized higher, though. It sticks you there, and helps pull you back up when you dip. Then you can gain more altitude and stabilize even higher, until you're where you want to be. You'll find more things you like come your way before too long.

You must appreciate every tiny lift, and every little gain. Appreciation accelerates your result—judgment and complaining reverses it. As you enjoy your way up, step-by-step, you'll stabilize so powerfully at each level that in the future, with a little attention to your Instrument Panel, you'll catch the slightest dip and maintain your altitude forever. Best of all, you get "rubberized"—you bounce off the bottom and snap back quickly. You can't be brought down for long.

At her second session, a client who had come to me sad and clinically depressed said she had some profound spiritual experiences the week after her first session. "Things got better, but now I'm frustrated and aggravated a lot." She was giving herself a hard time—here she was supposed to be getting better, and she thought this aggravation was a sign of something wrong. I suggested, "You came here depressed and in despair. Where is aggravation on your Instrument Panel? Look at it."

"Wow, I'm way up there at the halfway mark!"

"Yes, your nose is pointed in the right direction. You're at the tipping point. Stabilize there, just *be aggravated* for a while and then move on up. We judge certain emotions as bad, and they're *all good information.* Keep heading in a general upward direction toward more relief—that's all it takes. If you relax and allow yourself to feel what you authentically feel, Grace does the rest. Make it right, and let yourself dive into that aggravation deliberately, powerfully."

She immediately began to smile, feeling soothed. Soothing is what it's all about. Find that feeling of relief for yourself. Soothing points the nose upward. How would you talk soothingly to a child or a friend in need? "Oh, look, you're feeling a little bit better! Good for you! Keep going!" Do that for your self. To raise your altitude, talk soothingly to yourself until you feel a slight shift, not a dramatic shift. Just go for a little higher altitude. Step by step, and with the help of Grace, you can raise yourself to a very good place, and after wobbling a bit, stabilize eventually and stay up there.

I've never flown an airplane myself, but I've known enough pilots and watched enough movies to know that if you jerk the stick back and try to climb several thousand feet too quickly, you risk destabilizing your aircraft and crashing. By the same token, a steady ascent is easier on you, your life, your family, and your body. If you will attempt to gain just a little altitude each day, each week, each month, you will stabilize at each new altitude and maintain your gain permanently.

You've probably seen what happens when sudden fame strikes, and a person who is not accustomed to those heights can't maintain it, crashes, and melts down. Studies show that most people who win the lottery end up back where they started within a couple of years. The outer addition of money doesn't help, because they weren't vibrationally ready for it. It has been postulated that if all the money in the world were redistributed equally between everyone, within two years it would be back in the same hands it's in now. With no change in vibration about money, everyone would recreate their former state, for better or for worse. When all at once you try to fly higher than you're used to flying, too often it doesn't last. But when you rise gradually, Law of Attraction supports you and you stabilize at each new incremental level.

Contentment and boredom are actually nice resting places. There's a relaxing of tension that occurs at those points that is a great relief, which releases resistance. It's not yet up to hopefulness and it's nowhere near bliss, but it's on the way there. Again, rest—be happy you're up that far, and release resistance to where you are, which frees you to move up more. If you're coming up in altitude, and feel like doing nothing, do nothing—you'll feel different soon. Give the energy time to build. You're probably dog-tired from being in resistance for so long and need a break.

Practice choosing thoughts that raise your altitude on every topic in your life until it becomes a natural habit. Write your rises in altitude and other successes in your notebook until the resistant mind begins to get that *it is actually working.*

Your job is to release resistance to being who you really are, let go and let God, and let Grace in. Just set the intention to tip the nose of your plane up, and relax.

There's really only one question that's important as you climb:
Is the nose of my plane tipped up or down?

You Create What You Focus Upon

EVEN THOUGH DIVINE GRACE is lifting you up, you either use your Free Will to go with Grace or to resist it. Your attention is powerful. When you consistently focus upon what you want, it's like pointing the nose of your plane toward it. You end up where your nose is pointed. Focus on where you want to go and you arrive there, in time. Each time you detour (complain to yourself or friends, tip the nose down, talk about it not being here yet, indulge in negativity), simply point the nose toward your desired destination again (look for what's good, imagine you're there, tip the nose up, get in Large Self perspective), and soon you're back on track.

I live six miles from the airport as the crow flies. I can see it from here. But I have to drive fifteen miles to get there. There is no road straight through to the airport from my ranch. Life is like that sometimes. Just take the road you're guided to take and stay focused on the destination, not the indirect route. Even if you get off course, your Large Self, your internal GPS, recalculates your route, so you can't really fail as long as you keep moving.

When you consistently focus upon what you don't want, it's like saying you want to go to California, but then pointing the nose of your plane toward New York. Pointing toward New York, talking about how crowded and noisy New York is, thinking about New York, and complaining about how you keep ending up in New York keeps landing you in New York.

In life, focusing on what you don't want and expecting to get what you do want is insanity. Even though you have very real physical evidence of the unwanted reality, you can't afford to focus on that. Focus so intently on what you want that you drown out all contradictory vibrations. Then the essence of what you want *must* come. But don't get tense about *when* it's coming, or a specific form it must appear in—that increases resistance! Enjoy life, appreciate what's already here, and stay open to all possibilities—that reduces resistance.

Most humans keep looking at the unwanted thing and give their power away to it, unwittingly feeding it their energy. The wife is not doing what the husband wants her to, so he thinks about his dissatisfaction all the time. Her behavior magnifies from his attention to it, they fall out of love, and they divorce. Terrorism exists, so our leaders encourage us to fear it and focus on it, which increases our insecurity and fear. War is real, we don't like it, and we want it to go away. So we talk about how bad it is, we read about it, protest it, join groups who oppose it with us, and argue about which politician's fault it is. We become generators of aggression. The good news is that each of us affects the collective powerfully by raising our own consciousness. A highly enlightened person offsets and balances the collective consciousness energy of millions of lower vibration people. High vibrational energy is exponentially more powerful than the same amount of lower vibrational energy.

The nature of Life is constant change and everything in our lives is constantly moving. It never really stands still so you can turn it on a dime if you stop vibrating the same old thing. Disease would heal itself and money situations would improve naturally if we vibrated health and prosperity. When we obsessively look at disease and debt, we literally keep creating the same thing over and over again, because our attention feeds our own power to it. When you're hooked by something really strongly, notice you're pouring your gas into its tank, draining your fuel while fueling it.

After working with thousands of people, I noticed that most who were in therapy were constantly creating *more* issues and unpleasant feelings—*by talking about them*. Therapists, teach them to focus and feel. The Grace this book offers makes it easier, and many therapists use it who are committed to their clients becoming free and independent.

You're always "manifesting." The key is to know HOW you're doing it.

Sometimes people say, "But I need my outer reality or this person to change before I can feel good." I say "Uh-oh, you're in trouble now! That's backwards, and it strips you of your power." How empowered are you if your environment, other people, and outer circumstances can determine how you feel? When you choose your focus, no matter what is going on, no matter what anyone else is doing, no matter what your circumstances are—you are free. Claim your power to create whatever you want from wherever you find yourself. I want my nose tipped upward independent of what anybody else is doing or saying. When I'm up here, I can help others get up here, too.

Just on principle, don't let anyone cause you to feel any way that *you don't choose*. That's the most important power you have—to choose your attitude, and your altitude. Claim your power, and *decide* to keep your vibration up independent of everything else. Nothing is worth dropping your vibration.

The most famous, and most extreme example of this power to choose is detailed in Victor Frankel's book, *Man's Search for Meaning*. Frankel survived a Nazi concentration camp with his heart open. He determined that he would remain loving, care for others, remember his purpose, and keep his thoughts focused on living, even amid constant daily evidence of death, meaninglessness, and cruelty. His power to choose his reality remained intact. He influenced others to make this fundamental choice—to choose their own thoughts, their own feelings, and their own attitudes. He refused to hate his captors, so he never closed off *his flow of love* nor lost his alignment with God.

The key to creating what you want is to focus on what you want, then let go, and don't contradict it. Then the Law of Attraction must bring it to you. If the unwanted thought or reality grabs your focus again, quickly pivot. Good mantra: *Nothing* is worth lowering my vibration!

Think of your focus as a powerful laser beam that etches and carves your reality, and you'll be more deliberate about where you point it. Our website lets you hear samples of our uplifting original music collection: *Watch Where You Point That Thing*. A book by the same name is coming soon.

Don't fret about your lower thoughts and feelings—that just lowers your altitude! Your positive thoughts are more powerful than the negative ones, and the dominant force of Grace in the Universe is on your side. Don't worry. You only manifest seriously unpleasant things when you allow those low vibrations to simmer for quite some time.

Habitually happy people have consciously or unconsciously trained their biochemistry to be happy. Train your mind by practicing good-feeling thoughts. Say to yourself, "I will feel good no matter what." Be so dedicated to feeling good, and so committed to being in alignment with your Large Self, that you always find some way to feel just a little bit better in spite of *any* outer condition. What other sane choice is there?

Most people think when they describe a situation they're reporting facts. But when you describe it, you start vibrating it, then you're actively creating it. *Watch where you point that thing!* Your story about it creates vibration, and vibration creates reality. Be conscious of your stories, what you give your attention to, and what you create! When people tell their stories in sessions, I remind them, "It doesn't matter how much evidence you have that it's true. The only two things that matter are—does it point the nose up or down, and which way do you want to go?"

Soothe yourself. When you observe something you don't want, say, "Everything always works out. This is temporary. It will change. All I want is coming to me. Might as well feel better now, in the process."

Stop letting what you observe "out there" dictate your feelings. If you let "the facts" dictate your vibration you have no power—you're a victim. Be a creator rather than a reactor, observer, or reporter of "facts." Choose the way you feel and the reality you live in.

Others will not always understand your choice and may even accuse you of not caring for them if you won't commiserate with them, but you do the most good in your world when your altitude is highest. You cannot help anyone at all when you go down there. Let them know you love them, listen to what they say and feel, but don't go down there with them. I don't preach or teach outside of class. I just listen compassionately, nod, and shower them with love. But I don't go down there. People who want you to suffer with them may say, "You're being selfish!" With compassion and humor, you can say, "You want me to feel bad with you? Who's being selfish?"

Focus on what you want. Rave about what's right.

Dive In And Be With It

I ENCOURAGED YOU to tip the nose up, raise your altitude, and decide that feeling good is paramount. Now, this "dive in and be with it" piece I'll soon show you might seem paradoxical, or even contradictory. Step outside of black and white thinking, and you will see that there is an appropriate situation in which to use each method, and *they both lead to feeling good*.

"Tipping the nose up" and "diving in" each help you raise your vibration in different ways. Diving in is for your biggest challenges, for when you just have to go down and bounce off the bottom to come back up. Diving in raises vibration permanently. It frees you from *fear of feeling* in general.

The end goal of diving in *isn't to make feelings go away*. It's to feel feelings thoroughly in the moment, to return to that natural way of being children are born with. They feel every feeling, and it moves up, and they move on. You will relearn to let emotion move freely as it occurs, in the moment, as you are designed to do. When you reach enlightened equanimity, you will never suffer over feelings again. You'll allow them all, they'll all move quickly, and you'll bounce easily.

When you resist emotion, it drops down in vibration even more. If you keep resisting it, it goes underground. But it still vibrates down there and it still attracts things like it. When you just dive in and feel it, it quickly passes. It's so simple you will soon wonder why you didn't think of it all along. Therapists and Divine Openings Givers rave about how rapidly it works.

By diving in, I'm not talking about diving into the "story about the feeling." The story gets you stuck in the feeling, and generates more of the feeling, like running on a hamster wheel, and you'll actually feel worse. Drop the story; feel the feeling itself. Before you can fully experience the magic of "diving in," you'll need to know how to drop the story, and that's next.

What Story?

IT TAKES A WHILE to learn to even recognize our detrimental "stories." We've been telling ourselves these limiting stories unconsciously, and believing them to be "facts." They are not facts at all—they're interpretations and/or dramatizations. Intend to start hearing yourself think and talk.

For example, if you hate your job, you might talk to yourself like this as you drive to work: "I hate going to work. Why does it feel so bad? Hmmm, let's analyze where this feeling came from. It was my mother's domineering nature, etc., etc. … Should I tell them I quit? I shouldn't be feeling like this! I've been working on myself for twenty years! When am I ever going to just get a great job and stop having all this suffering? This job is holding me back. My co-workers are all so negative. But I can't quit because I'm afraid of having no job. This job is just awful."

Telling such a story to yourself or others, no matter how true you *think* it is, keeps you spinning on a hamster wheel and the emotion can't rise. Stories are the mind's interpretation, analysis and commentary. Stories are rarely a pure, objective, factual description of a situation. Stories justify and rationalize why you're right. Some stories set you up as the poor, good victim who has been wronged. The mind loves its stories—the problem is, they become your reality.

For better or worse, every vibration attracts more people, things, events, and feelings like it.

Stories actually increase any vibration, and keep you generating the same feelings and manifestations over and over. The pure fact is that *you have a feeling.*

It's all too easy to get caught up in a story "about" how wrong something was or is; the negative feeling is justified, fed, and it grows. The story holds you in the drama, and it doesn't resolve. You forget that you are the author of the story. The story is a trap you created.

It isn't always a "negative" story that holds you back. It can be an old positive story that served you at one time, but now doesn't. One client owned a mid-sized computer business, and for several sessions he struggled with attracting good employees. He had all the clients he needed, but couldn't find enough qualified people to service them. Of course we knew that his vibration was preventing him from finding good people, but couldn't isolate the vibration. I referred a brilliant unemployed technician friend to him, but interestingly, my brilliant friend kept finding excuses not to call him!

One day my client and I realized he had started his business with the belief that there were too many inept technicians out there fixing computers, and that his mission was to be the guy who did it right. This made him a very successful sole proprietor, but held him back from expanding—his old belief that he was the only qualified person was now working against him instead of serving him, as he kept attracting those inept technicians he had set out to save the world from, and repelled the good ones like my friend. He let it go and competent technicians started applying.

Another client's esteemed mentor had told him never to pay for work he could do himself. This was great when he had a whole karate school full of volunteer labor, but later, in another business, being the Lone Ranger exhausted him. One day he realized that story had to go so he could pay more people to grow his business.

We think we're describing reality, when we're actually creating reality.

The only important question to ask about any story or thought is, "Does it make you feel better or worse?" Whether it's "true" or not is not the point. Once you have an unhelpful story out of the way, the diving in process will work powerfully. It works by getting the energy moving. Energy wants to move. It was designed to move. It causes suffering when it doesn't move.

As you dive in, don't do it to "heal" feelings (they're not sick, they're valuable), nor to try to make them go away. When you don't let emotion/energy move, you create resistance in that area, on that subject. The frequency drops and becomes a low vibration in your body; Law of Attraction responds to what you vibrate and matches that vibration with more of the same. Let's say you feel anger at your mate, but you try to stuff it or go numb to it. It still hums quietly in you, attracting things you don't want, like anger from your mate, drivers on the road , or you stub your toe. Over time, you get progressively stronger signals. There's a physical tension, then a sensation, then pain. A dis-ease or some event could manifest to get your attention if you let it go on too long.

Many spiritual people try to do what I call the "spiritual bypass." They try to go from the lower vibrations straight up to love and peace. They'll tell me, "I try to surround the person I'm angry at with white light. It's not working." That energy-feeling vibration needs to be experienced fully. Feel the fear or anger or whatever it is, authentically. Then it will move. This can be done quietly in the privacy of your own mind. It is not recommended to act it out to the other person.

Two effective ways to bust out of a story.

1. **Tell yourself a better story** that moves you up the Altimeter. If that doesn't work:

2. **Use the Diving-In Process below.** It has you drop the old story altogether.

The Dive In And Be With It Process

This powerful step-by-step process raises even persistent lower feelings.

- Sit, close your eyes and give the *feeling* your attention. Imagine diving into it, or *soften and embrace it* like an old friend (which it is.)

- Drop the story and cast of characters, and feel the *feeling* underneath the story.

- Breathe for pleasure, letting your spine undulate gently. Breathe *softly* into the feeling, being very kind to yourself.

- Say "yes" to the *feeling*. This helps you *soften*. You might say, "I hate this feeling, but I will embrace it." Power is tied up in it, and fully feeling it gets your power back.

- Drop the story and all thoughts. If you can't stop thinking, repeat the above words.

- Feel your *body sensations*. You can name them: tight, warm, itchy, heavy, etc.

- Imagine the feeling is now just atoms vibrating in your body.

- Go deeper into it—*softly*. Breathe gently into it, like a baby breathes.

- Do not try to change it or make it go away—that adds resistance. Just feel it thoroughly.

- Once you feel even some relief, momentum will carry you upward. Relax.

- Open your eyes, notice how you feel. Claim your success.

ACTIVITY: Stop reading now and try it. Reading and mental activity don't change your life. People often say that on the second reading of the book, they realized they'd been merely in their head on the first reading. Experiencing, feeling, and moving energy changes your life permanently.

If the story is persistent and you can't drop it, get up and dive into the feeling as you demonstrate, move to, or dance to that feeling with your body. Then move yourself up through the feelings on the Instrument Panel. Raise your altitude slowly, step by step.

Diving In is one of the key processes in Divine Openings. Practice it until it's your new habit. Even after you've been happy for years, sailing along on a steady high, if your vibration plummets, the first reaction of the mind will probably be to make it W-R-O-N-G. "I should be beyond this now. I shouldn't feel this way." Making it wrong only compounds the resistance and prolongs your suffering. As soon as you can gather your wits, make it "right," value the message of those feelings, and experience them fully. You will rise, even from deep depths.

A couple of times I've said to myself out loud, "Pull it together, Lola. Let go—don't resist. It will rise." And it does every time! If you try to make it go away, want someone to "heal" it, or talk about it with you, you're giving your power away, and an opportunity to claim lost power is forfeited.

It's supposed to feel "bad" to be down there, and you can be sure that "bad" feeling points the way to a whole new freedom if you make it right. You may need to dive in more than once on the same subject if you can't let yourself feel it all at once, but soon you'll get it.

Once you get Diving In, you can use this shorthand version:

- Breathe softly into the feeling.

- Drop the story and feel the feeling.

- Experience the physical sensation.

- Feel it as vibration only.

- Breathe for pleasure while you be with it, in no rush for it to pass.

Drop the story. Feel the feeling.

The analogy of diving into the feeling as if it's a big pool of water makes it easier to remember to do this when you need it. Even when you know this effective strategy for finding relief, one of the hardest things, right in the middle of confusion or crisis, when your thinking is not at its sharpest, is to remember to do it.

During the twenty-one days of silence, I found that any feeling, fully experienced, appeared to dissolve. Now I know the energy rises to a higher frequency, and as it rises up the Instrument Panel, that power is reclaimed and becomes available for productive use.

If you feel numb, dive into the numbness, and that too will move and resolve. Although most times you can dive in and move a feeling quickly, there are times when you need to give yourself a day or two to be with it. If you dive in and it doesn't move, go about your business, letting yourself feel however you feel for a while. The less you make it wrong or resist, the faster it will rise.

Everything is vibration. It's atoms moving around. Breaking it down into pure and simple vibration, your experience of the feeling and the story might go more like this: "This is a feeling/vibration in my body," or "It's just atoms quivering. I can be with that."

Emotion creates a physical vibration, and by diving into it and experiencing it, you can let it move into a higher vibration. Pretty simple. No story, no suffering. Any emotion can be experienced like that, even if you don't like it. As you get better at this, you will begin to feel things purely in the moment with no verbal description, no story. You will vaguely identify the feeling or vibration and dive into it, and then it will move up. Soothe yourself by saying, "Everything vibrates. Notice how this vibration feels. Vibration wants to move."

ACTIVITY: Try experiencing everything as vibration in your body this week. Feel everything as atoms vibrating in your body without labelling it "good" or "bad." Drop the names for the feelings, ignore your mind's stories about *why you feel that way,* and for this week simply experience everything as flowing feelings. When you can experience pure vibration you'll get incredibly free and more psychic. Vibration is pre-feeling—you can feel it before there is even an emotion about it!

Diving gently into the feeling brings the power of your Divine Presence to the situation, lighting up new circuits, illuminating new choices. After you tune up your vibration, you'll be clear-minded and aligned with your powerful Large Self. Then if there is still any problem left, you'll let go and let The Divine do the heavy lifting, or you'll be guided what to do. Everything moves along more easily once there's no negative emotional charge on it.

If you experience difficulty diving in, or it doesn't resolve, order the ***Dive In And Be With It*** audio set online. It walks you through this key process as you relax. It's easier to let go because you don't have to think; you just lie down and let The Divine do the heavy lifting. It includes many types of diving in on various subjects. Never let yourself get stuck. This is *your life!*

Any feeling un-resisted moves, rises, and frees you.

As you dive into a feeling, you are "being with what is." That reduces resistance, and frees up the flow, providing instant relief. Even if it's only a little relief, you instantly know that the nose of the plane is now pointed upward, changing your trajectory. Even if you point the nose upward just a bit, that's enough—it makes all the difference in the world—you don't hit the ground!

With no story to keep regenerating the lower feeling-vibration, you will let go at some point. It is only energy, and when the pipes are opened, only love and bliss flow through. I have in ten minutes raised abject fear or deep grief into bliss.

A client, an attorney, came in with a million dollar lawsuit, two runaway teens, a recent divorce, and his business going south. Within an hour he was feeling better, and in two sessions he was feeling better than he had felt in years, although nothing had materially changed yet. He looked stunned, but felt better. This radically disrupted his reality. The mind thinks happiness is dependent on outer circumstances. Hey, anyone could be happy if everything and everyone around them was always like they wanted it. Mastery is choosing happiness independent of outer circumstances. He began an upward spiral after that, and his life opened up. Three years later he's doing his dream of working in the music business, regularly putting on shows. His most recent show starred—guess who? His two sons.

The feelings that give us the most difficulty are ones that we've resisted the longest. If it were just a momentary "now" feeling, it would not hook you or be such a big deal; it would flow on through you and upward, as feelings are designed to do, and it would be gone, never thought about again. When it sticks with you and won't move up, or if it recurs frequently, you know you have a long-practiced habit of resisting that feeling. There is a deep pool of similar vibration within you. A current situation can activate that old, well-practiced vibrational habit and make it seem as if all of that negative feeling is present right now, when in reality the bulk of it is from the past. It makes a current problem feel much bigger than it really is.

Remember this when you hit a really big pool of vibration. It's not happening today. It's old energy. Be with it, let Divine Grace raise that vibration, and you recover all of that giant pool of energy. When you can be with the feeling and let it move, you are free, and you are back in the moment. You're restored to your power as your altitude rises to the level where your Universal Source lives, which it naturally wants to do when we stop resisting. It's only our tensing up that keeps us low and creates distress. When we allow the feeling to flow, we return naturally to wellbeing every time.

Be patient with yourself on this if you have many years of practice telling your story. You'll build confidence and prove to yourself that diving in does work. You will over time retrain yourself to stay out of the story and just be with the feeling, and you'll go higher faster with each success. You'll catch yourself in a story and ask yourself, "Hmm, is this story productive? How does it make me feel? Where does it take me on the Instrument Panel? I'll feel this fully, and it will move."

Give yourself appreciation each time you use your Free Will choice, catch a story, and find even a little relief. You now know that what you focus on consistently over time, you create more of, so focus more on the good stuff, and move the lower feelings fast. The more you practice this mastery, the faster your fleeting lower vibrational emotions will rise to higher vibrations, and the more confidence you will build.

If, for example, you are having trouble losing weight, don't push against the weight or tell your story about how hard it is, or how you can't eat what you want. (It is obvious from looking around that what people eat isn't the whole cause of fat.) Dive into the *"fear of fat" feeling* and be with it till it rises. Slow metabolism is just suppressed, stagnant physical energy that's vibrating low. Be with the feeling, it will move, and new solutions always open up after that.

The same goes with money difficulties. Forget money itself (it's just a byproduct of your money vibration.) Dive into the *fear or worry about* money. Be with the feeling softly, not trying to change it, willing to face it without running. That energy begins to move, to rise in frequency, up the scale. Go for feeling better about "money and you" rather than dollars. It's easier and faster.

Authentic emotion is an infallible indicator of vibration. Pain and peace, bliss and anger are all made of the same Divine energy, but with different vibrational frequencies. Peace and bliss are energy that is flowing fully, and so their vibration is high and strong. Pain and anger are that same energy but pinched off partially, so their vibration is lower. Resistance lowers the vibration, slowing it down. Resisting emotions that feel bad only makes them slower, lower, and denser. Pain + resistance = suffering. What you resist *persists*.

Don't resist your resistance! Soften!

Unwanted emotions are just indicators that you're not vibrating the same as your Large Self on that subject. When you're feeling good, Divine energy is flowing through you freely. You're an open pipeline. It's supposed to feel bad to have your pipes obstructed and to be out of alignment with your Large Self. Be glad that it feels bad to be your small self. It's a reminder for you to let go, tip the nose up, or dive in, and get back to your Large Self.

Once the pipeline is opened, any emotion will automatically rise. Hurt, anger, and fear, after being experienced, rise to peace and bliss. It's all just energy—it only feels bad when we've resisted, clogged up the pipe, or further resisted it right into suffering.

To prove to you that diving in is not about fixing anything or working on yourself, but just a raising of vibration, try this: if you are already high on the Instrument Panel, dive into that good feeling, and it too rises. You go even higher. Do it for fun. Your creativity flowers, and your passion soars to new heights. You find new levels of love.

While for most there is an easy, sweet return to bliss, some of you will experience an intensification of unwanted feelings as the lower vibrations arise and are felt, especially if you believe nothing good comes without paying a price of pain! Some need to see something dramatic happen to know it's "working." Those who let it be easier are later surprised to find things just changed "for no apparent reason."

Divine Openings is so helpful because it re-attunes and holds you to such a high resonance with your Large Self that all else must move on up eventually. Any pain you feel while stagnant energy moves up is only a ghost from the past. You might feel the emotions now, as if they're happening now, but remember—it is not happening now! You are on your way to bliss and peace and you never have to go back unless you get sloppy with your Free Will choices.

It's often said that public speaking and heights are people's two greatest fears. From my vast experience, I'd put fear of feeling atop that list. But Divine Grace does ninety percent of the work for you when you let go. Do your ten percent: choose to stay awake.

The best news? The days of slogging through emotions and issues for years are over. Now, once you dive in and experience just a few deep, old emotions fully until they rise into neutral or even bliss, you are on the way to being free from suffering and bondage to *all* emotions *forever*. You still have an entire range of emotions, but they don't run you.

When you fear no emotion, you are free.

The natural outcome of practicing the "diving in" process is at some point, you will seldom need to do it formally anymore. Feelings will just flow easily and naturally on the spot, without having to stop and think about it. You stop resisting feeling entirely. It moves up, and then you feel better. Health, well-being, and prosperity are all about moving up vibrationally. Practice flowing emotional energy, then you can flow money energy, creative energy, and physical health energy better.

Should I Dive In, Or Tip Up The Nose Of The Plane?

ONE DAY A client asked, "How do you know when to dive into the emotion and experience it fully so that it rises, and when to just tip the nose up and change your thoughts?" One of these methods always works. Both end up with feeling better. Both have you value all feelings as messengers. Both teach you to let emotion and energy move freely.

Here is the distinction I use: if you've tried repeatedly to raise your altitude on a particular subject, and it doesn't stay up, dive in. There is probably a large stagnant pool of old, resisted feeling, a blind spot, or numbness. A feeling will also come back if you resume telling the old story and create it again.

We all pick up stories, habits of thinking, and beliefs by attuning to the energy of parents, teachers, society and others. Most of us have vibrational habits we don't know we have. It's on autopilot, and goes unnoticed. Notice your stories. Get Divine Openings sessions if you need help.

Anytime I feel anything less than good, I know that the small self has latched onto something contrary to what my Large Self feels about that. There's nothing to "do" except let go. When I can just be with it and let it move up it's that easy—only when I resist is it harder.

I am where I am, and compassion and acceptance of that reduces resistance, and relieves me of the need to work on myself anymore. As enlightenment unfolds, the small self might find sneaky, subtle ways to keep us in stress. Many months after my long silence I built up some physical tension after not having any for all those months, and asked The Indweller for insight.

Soon I had a dream in which I had been on a nice vacation and it was time to go home. I had left my baggage at the home airport on the way there. I had not missed it at all, but suddenly wanted it back when it was time to go home. I called to arrange the proper procedure to get my baggage back, and was suddenly feeling stressed. The feeling, tone, or vibration of a dream tells you more than the story line. My small self was saying, "OK, vacation over. I want the old familiar life back again." It didn't care that the old familiar life was way less fulfilling and wonderful. I woke knowing that my small self was bringing stress back into my life to get back to familiar territory. I had even started drinking caffeine again, which makes me tense. I don't need caffeine at all to be energized, so why was I using it again? I stopped. Relaxation returned.

With Divine Openings, dreams don't require analysis—even "bad" dreams are nothing to worry about—the dream is moving the energy for you. The rules change at different levels of consciousness. Just feel the dream, notice your intuitions, if any, and take any action that feels right.

I want to invite you into a big-picture perspective for a moment. This focus on emotions is going to pass, and you'll soon be living in a fresh, new reality with very little dramatic emotion. Tears are likely to be tears of joy. Once all the energy that used to be tied up in lower vibration is liberated, you begin using it to play and create—living fully—more powerful and free than you thought you could possibly be. Surprisingly, mastering your emotions is your ticket there. All the esoteric studies in the world can't bypass mastering your emotions.

Negative Manifestations That Still Show Up After You've Raised Your Altitude

FIRST OF ALL, everything that happens is valuable information, and calling it "negative" devalues it. Whatever is playing out for you right now is the perfect product of how you vibrated in the past. It's an echo of your past. If you're not creating that anymore, it's already history, and you can change your tomorrow right now. Appreciate it all and it changes faster.

In this physical world, things that exist in the material today are here simply because energy, thoughts, focus, and feelings (conscious or unconscious) from the past built up to a critical mass to create them. Today's reality is a product of weeks, months or years of that vibration.

Even when you raise your altitude today, some people, events, and things were already in the delivery truck on their way to you. It might (or might not) take a bit of time for the old manifestations to stop being delivered, and for the new things you want to get delivered. You can neutralize any old, pending manifestation right up to that point of momentum where they are already on the physical delivery truck on their way to you.

We think we want instant manifestation, but be grateful that there is a space/time lag before our thoughts manifest. Be glad a particular vibration has to occur consistently for some time before there's enough critical mass for it to show up in the physical. If there wasn't a lag, your slightest fear or worry would show up in front of you within seconds—you'd worry about being eaten by a shark, and presto, a shark, a pit bull, or a lawsuit would jump out and try to chew you up! Fortunately, in this dimension, the time lag allows us plenty of time to catch it and say, "Whoa, better tip the nose up and find a better feeling before something like this manifests!"

NOTE: You don't always manifest literally what you felt or thought about, but the vibration always matches. For example: resisting change and not owning responsibility for our reality attracts broken bones, they snap under the pressure. Feeling like the world isn't safe attracts victimization.

One client started having accidents right after we began our work together. First he sprained his ankle playing with kids. That triggered a worsened dependence on the painkillers and anti-depressants he came to me to get off of. Then the next week he fell down his stairs due to painkillers, and so "had to have" more painkillers! There are no accidents.

I had an "aha." "Were you always accident prone?" He indeed had an old belief that he was unlucky and life didn't support him—this was just an old vibrational habit. The good news is that with Divine Openings, what comes up is moving up for good. He rapidly got better and went on to kick the addictions that were ruining his marriage. Now he's a new dad, has a great job, marriage and life, and is doing his music.

His Large Self knew that there was an opportunity to get it all out on the table, and brought him just the incidents he needed to make sure he saw his vibrational habits. He seized the day and took his power back.

Besides feeling good and becoming free of slavery to the emotions and the mind, living in a higher vibration has a stunningly wonderful natural result. The more you live in higher vibration, the better the outer conditions go. If you encounter people and circumstances you are certain do not seem to match, then there is a vibration you are not aware of—I call them blind spots.

The only reason one would not recognize an incident as a natural product of one's own vibration is not being in touch with the feeling or vibration that generated it. Either they have learned to ignore it, numb it, rationalize it, or explain it away—or it has been in their body for so long, perhaps even since birth, that they don't notice or feel it. It's invisible and unconscious.

People become accustomed to a feeling and think it's normal. They have no other experience to compare it to. Unfortunately, we tend to adjust to the pain or lack in our lives, and think of it as normal. An abused child may beg to go back to the abusive parent—it's familiar—it's home.

In other cases, the person is not aware of how important it is to feel good, or they have been brainwashed by a society that doesn't value good feelings. They feel "bad" about choosing to feel good! How sad is that! Do you watch bad-feeling TV and movies, read bad news, and talk about horrible things with no regard for how it makes you feel, and what that creates? If you want something different, change your focus.

Imagine an airline pilot gazing ignoring the altitude reading on his Instrument Panel as the plane heads toward a mountain, or ignoring the low fuel reading until he runs out of gas.

But being conditioned as most of us were, we often did ignore our Instrument Panel. Or the feelings that were amped up by the stories became so painful we had to shut them off. We ran from, resisted, and tried to fix our painful feelings for so long we forgot how to take our own bearings. No one's blaming us for doing that. We just got separated from our own inner wisdom.

From birth onward, well-meaning people encouraged us to listen to them instead of our own feelings. School in particular was geared to teach us to conform and obey, to listen to outer guidance, not the inner voice, and to tone down our energy, go against our natural desires, and delay the gratification of our passions. So much of what we were taught was designed for the convenience and pleasure of others, not for our empowerment.

So it becomes that we don't know which way is "up" on the Instrument Panel. Some people's Instrument Panel got turned upside down and they thought feeling good was bad, and feeling bad was good. From now on, you'll know which way is up, and you'll come to know that it's simple: *good feels good, and bad feels bad.* There is a whooshing current of energy I feel every time a client catches that tailwind of their Large Self and begins to soar toward alignment with it. "Can you feel that?" I'll ask. Most can. They are remembering how to feel subtle energies they'd long ago become desensitized to. This return to feeling is the door to bliss.

Divine Openings move feelings and reconnects you with energies you've lost awareness of. Grace does for us what we cannot do for ourselves. Just stick with it and do your part—let go and get out of the way. Choose the highest vibration you can at any given moment. Say yes to every feeling, soften, and energy moves naturally.

Your Credit Rating

MY FRIEND WAS upset that he was still getting aggravated with his business partner. He said he had made no progress in keeping his altitude up despite all his efforts. "Hmm," I said, "That's not what I see from here. I see you getting way less upset than you used to. I see you holding your altitude much higher as you deal with it." His eyebrows went up as he realized this was true. Give yourself some credit. As you evolve, as you become accustomed to feeling good, you are going to become more acutely aware of even the slightest dip in your altitude. This is great, but it can cause you to judge that you're slipping backward when you're not really.

Let's say ten is the highest altitude possible, and in general, your old altitude used to average a five. Once you start flying higher most of the time, and get used to averaging a seven, feeling something in that old five range will now feel as awful as it used to feel to experience a three when five was your high. The five is now your "new low" when it used to be your high. It's all relative. But give yourself some credit—you're at five even when you're upset now! You used to live every single day at five, but you were accustomed to it. Now you're accustomed to higher. See how this can cause you to discredit yourself?

The mind is a wrong-seeking missile. You don't have to always listen to it.

One client astounded me when she rated every area of her life as at least an eight or nine on a scale of one to ten. She had one area she rated as an eight and it was really bothering her. Most clients put up with eights happily! They usually don't come to me until their average is much lower. But an eight felt to her like being really stuck in that area, since she was used to nines! Eights will feel *bad* to you when you get used to nines. Don't let your mind make the feeling wrong. It's valuable information. It's telling you how to get in even closer alignment to your Large Self.

Go easy on yourself. Where you are is where you are. There will always be contrasts, things you like better than others. Notice and claim that you are higher than ever before, that your lows are now higher than your highs used to be. The more you notice and appreciate how far you've come, the more the Universe can match that appreciation and bring you more things to appreciate. In the financial world "appreciation" means your money has compounded. It means the same thing in the vibrational world. Appreciation compounds your assets.

Make the most of the best and the least of the worst.

Of all the people in the world to set your relationship right with, you are your number one relationship, so appreciate yourself generously. Appreciation is the vibrational equivalent of love. We may not know how to "love ourselves more" in practical terms, but we can always find tangible things to *appreciate* about ourselves.

Every time I do something a little better than before, or any tiny little thing goes well, I hit my "Easy" button. It's a red button from Staples Office Supply. When you hit it, it says in a cheerful man's voice, "That was easy." By celebrating and appreciating every single thing, I create more to appreciate. Make the most of the best and the least of the worst, since we create more of what we focus upon. Appreciation is a magical act. Make a habit of giving yourself generous credit, plus some for good measure. Express your appreciation to yourself, everyone, and everything. Appreciation is an important part of the ten percent that's yours to do. If you were raised not to build yourself up, how's that been working out for you? If it's hard at first, adore The Presence within you—that's an easy way to start.

Divine Opening

CONTEMPLATE the photographic work of art for two minutes,
and then close your eyes and experience.

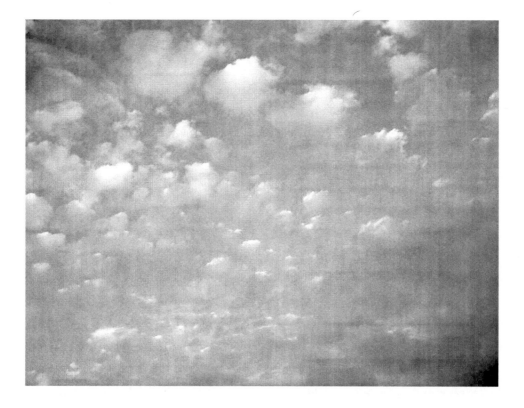

*Figure 8—**Light Clouds**, enhanced photograph by Lola Jones.*

All the art in this book is shown in color in the Art Gallery at www.DivineOpenings.com.

Seeing My Smaller Self

I DON'T RECOMMEND that you go looking for negativity in yourself, or anyone, *ever, at any time.* But you'll feel when you're vibrating lower because Divine Openings makes it increasingly *intolerable* to stay in lower vibrations. It will feel awful, and it should! Don't make it bad or wrong, don't be afraid of it or resist it. The vibration will rise with your loving, gentle Large Self embrace. There is nothing to do. The "bad" feeling plus the desire to feel better propels you toward what you want.

The darkness is not your true self. It's only what you experience when your smaller, denser self closes its eyes to the light. Embrace the small self, be with it, and soon, although you remain human and imperfect, you are not run by it anymore.

Our positive spiritual personas and pretensions are just as insidious as any negative personas. As I asked The Divine for relief from some false selves I had built up, I didn't like what I felt and saw, but was willing to be with it. Then as I naturally pivoted from what I didn't want to what I did want, a wave of strong desire to be more authentic washed over me. How had I not seen how false it was to pretend to be more cheerful than I really was? How had I not seen the degree of my alienation from other people? A transactional mentality showed itself. There was loss-prevention strategy in some of my decisions that made no sense in my rich and blessed life. I was kind to myself and didn't condemn, so those layers of masks fell off, leaving me tremendously relieved and renewed. In the light of consciousness, the vibration rose, without any work.

Once awakening begins, we are glad to see these things! My job was to relax and receive—and let the Divine do the heavy lifting. Lately, all I have to do is focus lightly on something I want, and it develops fairly quickly. There is no more working on myself. I'm on "automatic evolution," and you are too; as soon as you stop seeking and let it be this easy, the desire is often granted overnight. Appreciation poured out of me for yet another degree of freedom and authenticity. I'm still not perfect, and it's not about perfection, it's about the ever-unfolding, evolving journey.

There's no need to figure out or fix your human imperfection. Just gently be with it.

Emotions After Awakening

THE BEST NEWS is: as you become more expanded, you will have less and less difficulty keeping your altitude up. The only reason we ever had any difficulty with heavy feelings is that we'd resisted feeling them fully. We'd been taught they were bad. We'd diminished them, slowed them down, or stopped the flow altogether. We did anything to avoid painful feelings. I know, sometimes it hurt so much! We'd get stuck in them and they seemed to go on forever. Well, no more.

Once you routinely "dive into" every feeling you feel, it's experienced *fully* and rises quickly. As you practice, it becomes your habit. Feelings flow through you as they were designed to do, quickly, easily, without thought, analysis, or processing (it would serve you to stop using the word processing.) The cowgirl in me says, "Stop the infernal processing and just feel. Simple."

You live and feel fully. You allow everything to move through your life with no resistance to persons, events, or feelings. You still have the full range of emotions. There is still contrast. You still like some things more than others. You just don't get as hooked or suffer over it. This is equanimity. You use your emotions as the valuable Instrument Panel readings they are.

You still get angry, sad, disappointed, and frustrated from time to time, and as you fully experience each emotion, it relaxes upward again. The more time I spend at higher and higher vibrations, the more Law of Attraction holds me up there, and the more "rubberized" I get. I snap back up into the higher vibrations faster and easier each time—as if a rubber band connects me to the top of the Altimeter. The longer I vibrate up there, the stronger and thicker that rubber band gets. Even deep negative emotion can give way to bliss very quickly when we embrace it.

Five minutes of meditation now goes deeper than an hour used to. A quick moment to dip within and shift to Large Self perspective can bring quiet bliss, or set off peals of laughter.

Enlightenment is different from saintliness where you never get angry and you always have your halo on. The Dali Lama is known never to suffer fools or time-wasters; he'll walk out of the room, terminating the interview abruptly. I know one enlightened man who smokes cigars and drinks whiskey at times. You could even be an enlightened grouchy character who speaks bluntly, tells off-color jokes, and annoys people. Your uniqueness remains or even increases, and your perspective is valued; oneness does not mean sameness or uniformity. Enlightenment does not mean perfection. Please drop your old stereotypes and be *you*. This is a whole new world.

We come here for the full range of individual expressions this dimension offers.

The Evolution Of Who You Are

SIX MONTHS AFTER creating a more personal concept of God, I evolved into a state where I didn't feel God as separate from myself at all. It expanded from a mere concept to a real experience. I know I'm not *all* of what God is, but I'm part of God and one with God. So now my daily dialogue feels for all practical purposes like a talking with myself—my Larger Self. That's now normal. What stands out as odd now is the voice and feelings of my small self.

This can be disconcerting at first if you've spent a lifetime looking to "outside" authorities: parents, experts, leaders, doctors, and a God who is "out there," above and separate from you calling all the shots. If you're accustomed to being told what is right and wrong, what is good and bad, and what is the "best" course of action to take, it's like taking your training wheels off and riding the bike alone. But that fear is just the remnants of small-self perception. We are never alone or separate!

Becoming your own inner-guided authority is a spiritually mature stance to take. What if this life (and The Creator itself) is more experimental, unfinished, and adventurous than we believed, and welcomes your help creating the future, giving you carte blanche to do whatever you like, and eternity to try different things? That might make some people nervous, especially if they require rules and absolute black and white answers to everything, but for those of you on the leading edge, it's exhilarating.

The good news about Self Realization is that you are responsible for your entire reality.
The bad news about Self Realization is that you are responsible for your entire reality.

I'm joking. There is no bad news. When we let go to the Large Self, there is no burdensome responsibility to micro-manage or strategize our reality. We are carried by a Flow of Life that easily relieves us of much of the work and struggle. Once we take that first step to open our eyes and claim our power, and let go of the details, the rest is easy. Divine Intelligence orchestrates our lives. We still co-create it with our Free Will, and we still take action, but the more we let go of tension and resistance, the easier it goes. We still pick up the hammer and hit the nail, but our aim is true, we hit our own thumb less often, and life is fun.

It is true that when the small self gets hold of the concept that *it* is God, trouble ensues. But that is one of the risks of this game, and you can handle it. And if you crash and burn, no worries—get up and have another go at it. We are all far too serious about this game called Life.

How would you live if you were sure you couldn't lose?

A New Way To "Work"

IN THE ALL-TOO-SHORT story of the Garden of Eden, there was a time when Man lived in ease. Food grew on trees, life was easy, and there was no work. Whether you believe that particular story is literal or a metaphor, most people agree on one point: somewhere along the way, man went astray. And ever since then, through countless generations, many daily lives have been long chapters of struggle, toil, and conflict.

Take a moment to review the "plot" of all the movies you can think of, and you will find that almost all revolve around a problem or a long struggle, and after much difficulty our hero/heroine prevails over the challenges. Very short scene of happy hero. End of movie. Two hours of pain and struggle, fighting or conflict in great detail, with a short nod at the end to the "happily ever after," which we never actually get to see play out in detail, so we don't have much evidence that it exists. The respite is short in any case, and is followed by another sequel that resumes with more struggle and strife. Hero prevails, fade to black. And that's entertainment! Think about it! That's our conditioned unconscious expectation, and no one questions that we call that entertainment!

We're not conscious of how deeply we believe life is that way—a long struggle, with very short bouts of happiness. Some movies don't even give us the happy ending (those are considered the more "realistic" or "important" movies.) The Academy Awards favors those and snubs the happy, funny, "frivolous" movies. We don't notice these assumptions—we just live them. We don't have nearly as many role models for "happy most of the time" as we do for "strugglers and overcomers of hardship." The fascinating real life story of the racehorse Seabiscuit, the book, and the movie are all about overcoming crushing obstacles, with a little triumph and happiness sprinkled in here and there. And that's what we used to call "real life."

It's all right there in Technicolor in our movies. Rather than dwell further on how life lost its ease, let's skip right to the happy ending, which this time will not be short. The ancient story can change for you if you choose to shake off the mass hallucinations and create your own story.

The future you experience hinges upon the choices you make today. Reality is multi-dimensional, and every single person on this planet *experiences a different version of reality*. You really do live in a different reality than your parents, co-workers, or friends. We all have infinite potential, but some of us allow ourselves more possibilities, while others, to fit in and be comfortable, cling to the illusions and prescribed limits of consensus reality.

As you play with this more and more you'll notice that people act differently in the new realities you create. You and others look different in the new reality. Things work differently in the new reality. When people talk of doom and gloom—or this or that eminent global disaster—I'll say, "That's not *my* reality." I can't change everyone else's reality, but I can sure show them how.

For those who choose to claim their inner power, there will be an unlimited choice of realities. In the coming times work will consist of each of us doing what we were born to do, and enjoying it. Whether you are a truck driver, a hairstylist, a ditch digger, or a doctor, work will be an out-flowing of your genius and passion, an exercise in self-expression, a way to flow life force in a way you enjoy. You will play in this material reality, not to survive, but to create, experiment, savor, expand, and master your chosen endeavor. You will not spend your life making a living, which is survival, but making a life, which is creativity.

This return to The Garden is not an end goal. It is just another phase of evolution. We've entered a fast-moving new dimension of evolution that is unprecedented in recorded history.

The wooden plow is primitive compared to the giant combines of today. Today's fantastic reality was inconceivable to the medieval king. Similarly, we have no way of imagining from here what is coming. But it's fun to try—it stretches your sense of possibility and imagination! We will one day co-create even more fully with the Essence Of Life, not only on this Earth, but to create entirely new worlds in new dimensions. How would you like to be a "world designer"? You learn more about this in Level Two (it's all about joy and creating for the fun of it), and by Jumping The Matrix, which is essentially Level Three, you'll be playing with alternate realities outside of time and space. Most of the new developments go into those Online Retreat Courses because I enjoy multi-media— audios, videos, colorful graphics, art, and text are so easy to add to and update. The web is "alive," flexible, and perfect for the way I create.

Do what you love, and love what you do. It feels good flowing through you.

Life Proves Our Beliefs

WHEN A CLIENT lamented some manifestations he wasn't enjoying, he realized how his guardedness and defensiveness was bringing more manifestations that validated his belief in struggle, conflict and the need for guardedness. Each conflict validated his defensiveness and compounded his apparent need to be guarded. Life always brings us proof to what we believe is true. Then people say, "You can't just *pretend* it isn't true. See, it happened *again! Proof that it's real!*"

But a truth is only true because you believed it and collected big box of evidence for it, or a whole society believed it and you bought it. Then Law of Attraction made it truer.

It was understandable that his background as a martial artist had ingrained in him the need to be constantly wary of attack, and we talked about how that vibration had attracted so much discord with other people—lovers, business partners, friends. He saw it, but wasn't at all sure what to do. While it's usually easy for me to stay in cool, calm, Large Self perspective as I counsel clients, I got particularly plugged in after talking with him that day.

Soon it became clear why, and I received a gift of awareness too. Later that day, wells of tears began to flow out of me with the sudden recognition that I was somewhat defended too, but it just manifested differently with me; it was more hidden, and I didn't let the conflicts and guardedness show. I had played it out less overtly, and it was less damaging in my life, but it was there nevertheless. In facilitating clarity for him, I saw myself more clearly. I breathed easier on that soft, clear night as I let down the walls. I watched him become a little more open and less guarded with the world. His businesses thrived. My romantic relationship deepened. A friend who had harshly criticized me months before called and renewed our estranged friendship. Life opens more doors when our hearts soften.

Whatever you believe (and so vibrate) will repeatedly prove itself to you.

Boxes of Beliefs: What is "True"?

OUR MINDS AND bodies hold onto old vibrations, and boxes of evidence accumulate that "prove" our beliefs. We use our past experiences as our reference point for reality, to know what is true and real. There is a big problem with this. Any box of evidence you've collected is constantly attracting more evidence to prove it is true. You think life creates your beliefs, but actually your beliefs create your life. You think circumstances create your emotions, but that is backwards too— your emotions create your circumstances, and after a string of similar events you develop a belief.

If you believe people can't be trusted, that box of evidence actively attracts more people who can't be trusted. I don't have that box, and I rarely attract a person who can't be trusted. I am very trusting, but *discerning,* and it works for me. I accidentally left a purse with eight-hundred dollars cash in it in a disco in Mexico and got it back the next day. I've dropped fifty dollars on the floor of a store and had it turned in. I've taken rides from strangers. I constantly prove my box of evidence that I'm safe, and all I do is use my intuition wisely to avoid trouble. But that box works. No problem. What about boxes of evidence that limit you and cause you to judge others?

I used to have boxes of proof that I wasn't lovable. The experiences I used to have in relationships when I lived from that box now seem alien to me, although they were reality at one time. Now I feel completely lovable and secure, and am well loved; that's simply not an issue.

Everything is true—for someone, but it doesn't have to be true for you. I live in another reality now, outside that box. You wouldn't read a 1950s book about medicine or rocket science. The truths in your more expanded reality are "truer" than your old, more limiting truths.

Another example of this is a man with boxes full of evidence that his father was bad, and that extended to "males in authority are bad." The evidence may be factual and "true," but that box just attracts more abusive authorities. Such beliefs can ruin our lives without our understanding what is happening.

Some people have boxes of evidence that they are shy, or can't make money, or aren't attractive. Some have beliefs, supported by boxes of evidence, that they don't get guidance, or they are not smart, that the world is doomed, or that work is hard. I overheard a man in a coffee shop say, "That stuff about doing what you love and the money will follow—I tried it, and it's not true." I thought, "How sad. It's always been true for me. But he's right too, for himself."

Once you bust the box, you can just let go to the flow. The new paradigm has us receive the guidance or information we need in the moment that it is needed. You don't need boxes, just as you don't need prior experience of a route to take a trip. Just tune into your Instrument Panel and follow your guidance moment by moment. The mind wants boxes of proof, evidence, for security, but now you know it's deceptive. You don't even need "faith" with your Large Self to guide you. *Live in the now, not from boxes.*

Please relax around all this if you have any boxes that feel too big to bust by yourself. Just ask your Large Self to do it, relax, and let it happen. Grace makes all things possible—even things we have struggled with for years.

ACTIVITY: How many boxes of "true evidence" do you have that aren't helping you? In your notebook, write some things you believe that limit you, and ask for Divine help in letting go of that evidence.

How Do You Know What Is "Possible"?

How do you know if something is "possible" or "impossible" for you? Do you refer to the Internet, books, science, statistics, and your boxes? That's how most people decide if something is possible or impossible for them or anyone. Cancer? AIDS? Oh, that's incurable. Blindness? Incurable. Be prosperous? No way. Living simply? Not possible for me. Everyone on the planet being fed? Nope, there is only so much to go around.

If you have never experienced it before, or have never seen anyone on the planet do it, all the data in your boxes might say, "No, you can't do that, it is impossible," when Divine guidance might say, "Go for it, you can do it." How can we evolve above and beyond what's ever been done if we must have evidence that something is possible? This reinforces how important it is to give more credence to our own visions than to outer evidence boxes and past experience.

The earth is round, man can fly, the four-minute mile, talk to people halfway around the world—all these were once impossible, and that was backed up by the best science of the day. Now they're not only possible, they're *mundane*. For more on beliefs and freedom from them, search at www.DivineOpenings.com for the article, "Reality: Some Dis-Assembly Required."

Give over to your Large Self anything that is too big for your small self.

Give Your To-Do List To God

I STILL MAKE to-do lists and vision boards, but it's very different now. I think of it as putting it on the "God list" as one client dubbed it. Then I only do what I feel moved, inspired, and pulled to do, or must do for a deadline, like pay bills. Once it's on the "God list" it's done in the non-physical. Then I put it away and forget it! Instead of making myself do the items on my list, I stay tuned for inspired thoughts or urges to act, which for me are abundant. I love accomplishing things. If I think something needs action, I feel the vibration and check if it feels "ripe" or "cooked." I don't do much until I feel the tailwind behind it or even pushing it. If it feels sluggish it's not time yet, and no amount of action will make it successful. If the energy isn't cooked yet, action is wasted. When my energy is aligned with my Large Self on that subject, it's time to act.

I love it for big projects, big challenges, finding someone to do things I don't do well, creating money, finding just the right item, and receiving solutions to things I have no idea how to handle. I put all the mundane things as well as the "too big for me to handle" things on the mental God list. If I'm feeling resistant, I put it on *paper*. It is very efficient. A lot of the heavy lifting gets done by the Universe, by someone else, or it ends up not really needing to be done at all. Something often comes along that works better with less effort than you thought.

Let The Divine do the heavy lifting.

ACTIVITY: You might write on the blank pages at the back of this book.

1. Make a list of all the people with whom you think it is impossible to resolve issues. Then let go.

2. Write a list of things "too big" or complicated for you to accomplish, then let go.

Anything is possible for your Large Self. Just give it over and let go.

Where Does Action Come In?

THIS BOOK IS about tuning in to your inner guidance and becoming free from the incessant search for outside answers, but once you're tapped in, it's still a physical world you're operating in. Don't just sit at your desk and expect everything to come to you from within, or for free, although it might. We are interdependent and physical beings on this planet. That's part of the game.

Yes, some action is required to create in this world. This is a physical dimension. We came here to manipulate matter, communicate with other people, and create physical things, and we enjoy it. If we'd wanted just to create in the non-physical realms where everything appears instantly with just a thought, we'd have stayed in the non-physical.

Here, part of the game is material manifestation. It does get easier when we realize that 99.9 percent of creation is done with energy, focus, and intention, and that only that last one percent is physical manifestation. We waste less action and have more fun with the material action part.

I've spent all this time with you on the energy part. Now for the last part: action. Once your energy is up, and you're allowing the Flow of Life to carry you along, you'll feel inspired to act. Once you get clear on your true, authentic direction, a fire lights under you, compelling you to take action. You may be led to one step at a time. Begin by taking one step.

You came here to play in the physical world, to mold the physical clay. But it can be easier and more fun if your Large Self inspires your actions. People say writing is hard, yet I find it exhilarating, effortless, and flowing. I love writing and often can't stop. My Large Self does the writing. I read my own work and get reminded and inspired because it comes from a place larger than the small me. I let go and let it work through me.

You've said what you want. Now The Indweller, God, The Divine, your Large Self, whatever you call it, will give you guidance and lead you to what you need to do. You will be nudged in the direction of the people who have the skills and information you don't have—the great babysitter, the best accountant, the supplies you need, the best vacation deal, or the person who builds you a website that does a lot of the work for you.

One of those found me! Lee took a live Divine Openings Level One with his wife Brooke. I didn't even know he did websites, and he didn't know I was looking for a new one. A month later, he emailed me with a proposed plan for the exact website that I'd been shopping for. He proposed we trade the Five-Day Silent Retreat for himself and his wife. We started that week. Within two months I had an incredibly sophisticated new website, and within four months it was doing ninety percent of my work for me. Things started going *even better* in my absence!

Life brings you opportunities to co-create with others to accomplish goals, have fun, exercise, build a company, or tune up your car. It prompts you on the perfect timing to clean up a relationship, say hello to a stranger, make the phone call, hire the person, read the article, and follow the trail. It will seem like the most natural next step once the energy is lined up.

Your job is to tune in, feel the timing, and then take the guided physical action. I feel what I call a "smoothness" when it's time to act. It feels good in my body. The doubts aren't there.

You'll be guided. Just stay tuned in.

Follow The Guidance You Get

ONE CLIENT, who ended up being initiated to give Divine Openings, had huge awakenings after her first session. A hairball or two were coughed up. In the first week, awful recurring scenarios popped into her head where people she didn't know were abusing her or trying to control her. In her long-practiced habit of "spiritual bypassing" instead of feeling, she tried to "wrap them in white light and make them go away." They kept coming back.

As we talked about it, I intuited that she had not been allowed to express anger as a child. For all her life, when someone made her feel powerless, she could not let herself use anger to blast up the Altimeter. She had been trying in vain all her life to do the spiritual bypass on her negative feelings. "Just think love and light." Well, that's too big a jump from powerless to love, and most people can't make it stick. They fall back down, and then feel like they failed.

I had her dive into the experience, be with the feelings, starting from powerlessness, then move on up through anger. I coached her to face the abusers in her own mind, get angry, and tell them they could *not* abuse and control her anymore! Relief quickly followed.

Then I guided her to feel the feelings to the core, but drop the characters and the story. They had served their purpose. I led her through the diving in process. The feelings rose in vibration, and the "abusers" stopped appearing. Then she was authentically up in love, light and power, and could stay there.

Spiritual people sometimes, wanting to "be good," don't want to *ever* have, admit, or feel the lower vibrations, thinking that's failure. I see highly advanced spiritual people held back until they learn to embrace, allow, and flow their emotions. Once you embrace them, you rise out of them.

The main point of my sharing this story, though, is that those visions were her Divine guidance. We're looking for angels and listening for the booming voice of God, but from powerlessness, what God sends you is the impetus to get angry to get your power back. Once she knew that, she not only felt great—she trusted that negative feelings have a purpose. She began to honor and move them, not try to make them go away.

At the third session, I knew that the next level was about to pop. She was so revved up, she was running ninety miles an hour. Usually over-revved people are running from something, and it's usually feelings. My sense was that she had been running ahead of her body all her life. And who can blame her? Who would want to tackle something they don't know how to handle? But now you can do it with help from Grace. I soothed her, and she was ready to share that there was abuse in her childhood. She had been learning to dive in and be with it, but this subject was still daunting. So I guided her through simply feeling it, not analyzing it or telling the story, and the old, dreaded emotion was soon, as she described it, a pile of ashes. Once again, she was ecstatic.

That time her guidance had led her to me for help. From now on, with all that success under her belt, she'll be more able to dive into feelings and do it on her own.

Guidance doesn't always sound like you expect it to. It might take you to pain, or to an emotion or action that ultimately leads you upwards on the Instrument Panel. Follow it. It may not take you straight to ecstasy, but you'll certainly be on your way. You still have Free Will, and you can choose to allow the emotions, and take the actions—easily, or harder if you resist or make it wrong.

Guidance will look and sound different depending on where you are on Instrument Panel.
It will always call you upward, never downward.

Inspired Action

INSPIRED ACTION IS incredibly efficient. One hour of inspired action replaces thousands of hours of busy-I-should-do-this-hard-work-action. Now of course if you're building a stone fireplace, you still have to pick up stones and put the mortar between them. But if you're in inspired action you'll thrill to the physical movement, the newly forming creation, and the sore muscles. You came here to build with stones and mortar, to juggle numbers, and wash dishes, not to float in the ethers. Enjoy delicious action. And when the feeling changes, take a break.

How do you know when an action that comes to mind is inspired? When the mind is quiet and peaceful most of the time, just about anything that comes in and feels good is inspired thought. Remember, the voice of The Divine sounds just like yours, only smarter. Most of my thoughts are inspired, guided, nurturing, or uplifting now. The rest of the time my mind is not that active. When thoughts do run to the negative, I pay no attention to them, or turn away from, redirecting to the direction I want to go. At a certain point, you hear almost nothing inside. That's good! Don't run back to seeking and start all over again!

I compare my old mind to a cluttered airport runway with trash all over it. Your Large Self is always dropping packages on the runway, sending guidance. But the runway is so cluttered with junk we can't find the valuable packages in all the garbage. In the past I would muck around in the mind-garbage on the runway, not being able to decide what was valuable, and would get confused. The random, useless, mediocre or negative small-self thoughts were so abundant.

I'm very creative, and I always had so many ideas. There were so many potential things to do, and so many actions would come to mind. I would scatter my efforts too much, do too much action for too little result, or give up and do nothing. All that action kept me tired.

Once Divine Openings cleared the clutter off the runway, it was different. When a Divine inspiration came in for a landing, it was easy to spot it out there all alone, and there was no doubt whatsoever if it was an "important" idea or action. Now I know exactly which ones are the inspired ideas. They stand out like neon signs on that clear funway… runway. (Interesting typo—I decided to leave it in there.) No questions.

Even when my mind is busy, when my altitude is high, it's all high quality stuff, and I listen to it. A busy mind can be very productive. If you get too many thoughts to do all at once, write them down to capture them, then put them away. The timing will come to do them, or the Universe will do much of it for you, *or you'll get the result you wanted without doing anything.*

If the guidance is not clear and I'm not inspired, I don't act unless it's absolutely essential. I wait until all the pieces show up, and they do. I pay the bills and taxes on time whether I'm inspired or not, of course, but in matters where I have choice of timing, if there is confusion, resistance, or I'm not feeling good about it, I don't act or make decisions until there is clarity and inspiration. Uninspired action from the small self, without alignment with Large Self, is often futile, wasted action. Money, time, and energy thrown at a project out of fear or need are wasted.

Often when we're low on the Instrument Panel when we think about a task, that's a message saying, "Raise altitude before action!" We need to align with our Large Self and get to the party before jumping into action. Motivational speakers tell us to take massive action. We already work longer hours than we have at any time in recent history, thinking that more action equals more results, more money, thus feeling better. A quick look at the richest and poorest people in the world will tell you more work doesn't necessarily equal more money. Then again, when your action is inspired and you love the work, it's magically effective!

When you create your life in the easier "go with the tailwind" way, you may not receive much support from people who are out there working themselves to death. They may call you lazy, but you simply cannot please everyone. Let them do it their way. Do what feels right for you, and things will go much more smoothly. The old Puritan work ethic says work and suffering are virtuous. The "joy ethic" says work because it feels good, produce because it's satisfying, act when you're in alignment with your Large Self, and get to the party that's already laid out for you!

Procrastination or sluggishness is often your Large Self telling you that your energy is not yet lined up to your Large Self's level on the subject at hand, so why waste the action? When your resistance on that subject has relaxed and your altitude on it is high, you will suddenly feel energized and compelled to do some action, and it will work much better. This is letting go and letting God. Not everything has to be done this instant. That's your small self's judgment, some parental voice, or some goal-setting book you've read. So much of that stuff is contradictory to Divine Openings. Work, even hard work, is exhilarating when you're in the flow.

So, act, yes. But get your altitude up and point the nose where you want to go first with your energy. Otherwise you're flying into a headwind. You can't buck the natural forces of the Universe. It just makes you tired. Are you doing what your heart desires or are you following someone else's idea of "success"? Relax, listen, and get yourself to the party first.

Action and sweat can be rewarding. If it's not, look at where you might be out of alignment with your Large Self. The action that feels heavy right now may feel light once you've raised your altitude. Change your attitude toward it. Find some joy in it (EN-joy it.) Get yourself to the party; things look and feel different from there. It's a different dimension, literally.

In the midst of action, if you begin to slide down the Altimeter or grind your gears—STOP. Relax, take a break, release resistance, and re-align your energy. Tip the nose up and point it where you want to go. Stop looking at the obstacles. Reset your course toward your desire.

Give the big tasks over to God, let go, and wait for guidance. Go do something that feels good, and you'll return to the task refreshed. Forgetting it for a while releases resistance.

Our live and online retreats go much deeper into business and money. You can play there, with attention to your specific goals and challenges, and it is fun to be with others who share your vibration and celebrate your progress.

Energy, intention, and alignment pave the way. Action just follows that paved path.

Be OK With Where You Are

RELEASE RESISTANCE by making peace with where you are now. Say to yourself things like, "I am where I am! Where else could I be? Today is the product of yesterday's altitude. Tomorrow is the product of today's feelings, intentions, actions, dreams and visions."

You are where you are, and wherever you are is OK, because now you know how to get anywhere you want to go! Feel the instant relief in that?

Enlightenment is remembering your true essence that you're playing hide and seek from. As you open up to receive more Grace, you can remember and sustain that. Decide today to be all right with who and where you are. The Divine sees you as perfect, although evolving, right now. Each time you get impatient with a plateau, or bored with your old successes, stop and make peace with where you are right now. It's a form of being with it. Be with the fact that you don't like where you are, but lighten up on yourself. There will always be more you want.

Being mad at yourself is far more damaging than being mad at someone else. Your Large Self is never mad at you, so if you are, you are not aligned with your Large Self. If you must get mad, get mad at something or someone, or even God (who can take it.) It gives you the energy to move on up and reclaim your full power! Don't stop for long at anger, though. Keep moving!

Embracing where you are actually speeds your progress. The moment you stop making yourself wrong, your movement is freed up. You are no longer stuck. You can sail on much easier.

Soothe yourself.
You are where you are, and now you know where you are!

Questions People Ask

THERE ARE MORE on the website at www.DivineOpenings.com on the Ask Lola page.

I'm afraid I'll become addicted to this. Yeah, some people even get addicted to twelve-step programs. But the reason those programs work so well is that they show you that all addictions are just a misdirected search for spiritual bliss. If you get addicted to God's love, that's the real thing—it's healthy like being addicted to good food. You can go inward, get quiet and experience this energy anytime. You don't need a Divine Opening to get there once you've found that relationship within, so you won't get dependent on us. Keep coming for vibrational support until you don't need it.

I can't just become enlightened through this experience without doing the hard work on myself to get through my own fears, beliefs, and blocks. Do the practices, let go and receive the Grace. Let The Divine do the heavy lifting. That it has to be hard is the old paradigm. You can let that go now.

I wonder if this first time experience was the biggest high I will ever get, and will I be disappointed at future Divine Openings. Every experience will be different, yes. It will ebb and flow like the tides. It is cumulative, and does grow deeper over time. You cannot predict when the peak experiences, the cosmic experiences, bliss, or laughter will come. Enjoy each for what it is, then let them go.

How can I feel better when this moment sucks? Well, my dear, it is your response to this moment that creates your tomorrow. You simply cannot afford to focus for too long on what you don't want, what went wrong, or how awful it is. Sure, you are justified in your attitude; everyone will validate you. But the cost of dwelling in that justified victimhood is just *too high*. Don't let circumstances and people be your "excuse" for staying down, and not aligned with your Large Self. Pivot your thoughts from what went wrong to what you want, over and over. Or dive in until it rises. Choose power over powerlessness. Choose happiness over being right.

How do people get good things when they don't appear to be feeling good? He's mean to his employees, and he has a great girlfriend, and he's rich! It ain't fair! Well-being and abundant flow is the natural state of the universe. God loves all of you—you are one with God. Good things are always flowing to you and everyone else, without judgment, from God's Grace. Somehow that guy is letting that good in. Even when your altitude is low, God looks for every little crack of least resistance, every opportunity to give you your good. Judging those who have it actually slows it down in coming to you, not because you're "bad," but because your Large Self doesn't judge, so you're out of alignment with your Large Self. If you're in victim mode, you're not in receiving mode.

You can never know how that guy feels inside. Pay attention to how you feel. Look at your own Instrument Panel. You can know that. It's not so much that you need to work to create more of what you want; you just need to stop resisting the flow of good, the dominant energy of the Universe. You can let it in or resist it. Get out of the way! Forget about trying to figure out why people you judge as bad have the goodies. You can't read their Altimeter, and it's none of your business! You can't feel what's inside them and know what they're thinking and vibrating; it's "relative," it doesn't always show on the outside, and their words don't tell the whole story. They can sound grumpy but have a great money vibration. They can look and talk positive and seem all spiritual and yet have a terrible money or love vibration.

Judging people with money, or judging how they use it lowers your altitude and slows you down. Envy is a low vibration that shrinks your pipes and slows the flow of good to you. Just focus on your own vibration. Mind your own business.

The Divine has given you many good things (like Life) and is always looking for an opening to give you more. The Divine even uses your sleep time to bring you what you need, since during sleep you expand to your Large Self and relax into non-resistance. You go back to Divine Love and refresh and recharge in pure positive energy. A lot of good is allowed into your life during that rest as you let go and release resistance. That's why you feel good after sleep or meditation. Ever notice you usually feel better after resting, and circumstances improve? You always feel good as you wake. But if your normal waking altitude is lower than your Large Self's altitude, as you slide back to your lower altitude set point milliseconds *after* waking, you feel less good as you fully wake up. Notice this next time you wake.

Life is on your side. Will you be on your side too?

The "It's Not Here Yet" Syndrome

YOU WOULD RECEIVE everything you want—and enjoy the ride there—if you would just relax, let go of the past, and let the tail wind take you. All that you want would come in time. And each time you say, "It's not here yet," it is delayed, because you have vibrated in opposition to what you want. You have sent the delivery truck back to the warehouse. Don't even take score when the score is not in your favor. Take score only when the score is in your favor.

Whether it's enlightenment, more love, a wonderful home, or a dream job, the best way to let it come more quickly is by appreciating any part of it that you already have. If you want a lover, think of all the other types of love you already have, or remember the best parts of past loves, and feel it. Then Life can match you up with more of it. If you can't find any love in your past to feel, there's a clue. All your active vibrations are dominated by the "bad" feelings about your exes and your past. That's why you don't have love now. Or else other things are more important to you, you're splitting your intentions, and you just don't realize it. You may want your freedom and you believe love will curtail it. If you want your freedom very powerfully, freedom wins out.

You can want something too "badly." If you spent all day daydreaming pleasantly about only the having of it, it would come. But if you're feeing "bad" about not having it, you are creating not having it. The more you feel the *lack* of it, the longer it is in coming. If you radiate lack energy Life matches it with more lack. If you can't want it in a "good" way, just don't think about it at all. Do something else. That releases resistance too.

If you're working too hard on anything, take a break from it and do not think about it. If you want a great job, focus every day on the best parts of your current job. Appreciate your current job. "I do love working with Joan." "The hours are nice."

Savor the waiting for it. Start saying *(and feeling),* "I feel it coming." "It's almost here." "Won't it be nice when it's here? What will it be like?"

Don't take score too soon. Only take score when the score is in your favor. If it's not in your favor, delay taking score.

Daydream about the new job. It doesn't matter whether you imagine it, try new jobs, or remember past good jobs, you will create it faster if you feel like you already have it. Lack attracts lack. Abundance attracts abundance. That's why the rich get richer and the poor get poorer, unfortunately. Skew the score. Find evidence that it's coming, and delete evidence that it isn't. Most of the quality of your day-to-day life will depend on what you focus on. So next time you find yourself observing that it isn't here yet, pivot to what you do have, and feel appreciation for it.

Look for every opportunity to create love, humor, fun, and adventure. Radiate that, take steps toward it, and then let it in! That will work out a whole lot better than lamenting it isn't here.

And as always, if you can't just raise your altitude, dive into the lower feeling, or fear of never having it, until it moves up. You might use the Dive In And Be With It audio series to help you with this. You may have to stick with it until it moves, or do the process repeatedly for a few days, a little at a time—or it may move in one sitting. But as soon as it becomes work, let it go for a week. Go live!

I'm Not Resistant!

NO ONE INTENDS to be resistant or have a low vibration. No one intends to be unhappy. If you are still unhappy and your life is not working as well as you'd like, even after reading this book, there is still hope, if you read it again. Your freedom hinges primarily on your willingness to feel. I'll share with you here a training letter I wrote to the Divine Openings Givers:

"People who have difficulty allowing feeling struggle longer before they let Divine Openings help them. Because they've resisted feeling for so long, huge amounts of emotion try to rise, and it scares them. It's astounding to find that feeling is one of the most feared experiences on the planet. *Any feeling is a valuable message from your guidance system!*

One participant experienced his full power and God Self during the initiation in the Five-Day Silent Retreat. He felt he was about to levitate as he stood there, basking in the energy. Then a few days later he had a *huge* movement of old, stagnant energy (fear, terror, sadness, grief) accompanied by intense physical spasms, and he thought he was going to die! Having relied on "human strength" for thirty-five years, he didn't realize how much he had resisted feeling. He'd been doing Divine Openings, while resisting it, for two years—a superhuman feat! Holding back takes a tremendous amount of your energy. He realized why he'd been so tired. But the eventual and inevitable awakening of the True Self within pushes up anything that is not in alignment with it. Bliss tends to bring up its opposite and push out anything that is not bliss. Then that lower feeling rises. That's part of bringing it down to Earth. That may take a while (it doesn't have to) and can play out like old things blowing up (but it doesn't have to if you'll just feel.)

Men sometimes have more difficulty with feeling deeply, having been trained their whole lives not to show "weakness." What a handicap, having much of one's own Instrument Panel be off limits! For a man, anger might be OK, where sadness or tears are not allowed.

A war hero who fears no gun, bomb, or knife might break down into a twitching, terrified blob when confronted with his own feelings, or the illness of a parent or child. That feeling can't be shot, stabbed, or conquered, but resisting it only causes suffering.

Being around me is intense. There's a powerful, accelerated, evolution-inducing vortex that causes energy and feelings to move. I love it, but some romantic and work partners who were in strong resistance and didn't wish to feel and evolve simply couldn't remain in this field of resonance. Some actually melted down and had to get away.

Sometimes people attempt to manage everything with the mind, from the neck up, to avoid feeling. They try to think through feelings, or do the spiritual bypass and not have them. One man who is very, very powerful and successful in the world fled one of my courses in cold sweats with his back muscles completely seized up. Feeling had admittedly been his Waterloo through many phone sessions. I know he will complete the course when he's ready. He's a lovely, generous, sensitive person. He wants to make a difference, and does. This just demonstrates how terrifying it is to feel when the mind has told you for decades that you must not feel THAT! Anything but that!

Yet once we let go and feel it, we're FREE! Very quickly! People who commit and let go do not have these difficulties—Grace gives you a sweet, easy, lovely unfolding. But you need to know what can happen if resistance is stronger than you were aware of. You're not losing your mind, and you're not dying. (Some medical alarms do need attention.)

If it's tough, give it over to The Presence. It is truly not your job to do it alone. You asked for change, Divine Openings brings it.

Let it be easy. You get zero extra points for doing it the hard way.

Be assured that Divine Openings doesn't bring up anything that wasn't already there. It doesn't create a problem that didn't already exist. It only makes you aware of it so that it can move.

Read the book again if the first reading doesn't get you there. Many people really get it more powerfully on the subsequent readings, because Grace has softened and worked on you in the meantime, and you're more awake. While many of you are noticing big shifts by now, the next page offers more insight into how to let go.

Here are some clues that you might be unconsciously "prohibiting feeling":

- You analyze, rationalize, or think everything through instead of feeling it through.

- You get blindsided and surprised by people and events. You couldn't feel your Instrument Panel readings so you didn't know it was coming.

- You run around a lot, always in a hurry, rarely sit still, and stay constantly busy.

- Or you have low energy and don't get much done. You're tired, heavy, and weary a lot from holding back all that feeling that wants to move. Your metabolism is slow.

- Numbness. You're not sure what you feel on some subjects.

- You talk a lot. Talking is addictive for you.

- You have to be with people all the time, and can't be happy alone.

- Or you avoid people or intimacy, and have shallow relationships.

- You're always cheerful, but things don't go well. If so, the cheer is inauthentic and not what you're really feeling inside. You have blind spots—vibrations you're unaware of.

- You're cynical or resigned, or you settle for less than you really want.

- You act tough and you get treated tough by other people and by life.

- Or you get more "spiritual," and try to go around the feelings with positive thinking, meditation, spiritual bypass, or other means.

What if you suspect you're not feeling as much as you could? Be incredibly kind to yourself. Treat yourself like a sweet, precious newborn. Don't judge yourself—you got trained not to feel. It's not your fault. It's not "bad," it just doesn't lead to happiness, but you're going to be fine now.

Do the Daily Pleasure Practices and Thirty Ways To Raise Your Altitude from the end of the book. Take an "online retreat," watch the videos, and listen to the audios to immerse yourself in this higher vibration. Attend a live Divine Openings retreat. Demonstrate your intentions and commitments to yourself with action. Ask to feel. Then be willing to feel.

Divine Openings makes life easier pretty quickly, and the fun starts. It is not endless work. If you feel like it's work *at all,* you've dragged the old "endless work and processing paradigm" *into it.* Step back and enjoy rather than working on it. Just pay attention and make conscious choices daily

Some need one-to-one sessions or a live course to break through deep numbness, or if the resistance is very strong, the blind spot is big, or the mind is very dominating. It's your choice. Be kind to yourself and get the help you need. Some people take better care of their cars or homes or pets than themselves.

There are now Divine Openings Givers in more areas, and phone sessions are quite powerful as well, since Divine Openings transcends time and space. See www.DivineOpenings.com to contact me or other Divine Openings Givers.

Divine Opening

CONTEMPLATE the work of art for two minutes, then close your eyes and experience for fifteen or more minutes. Appreciate The Essence Of Life in you for your opening.

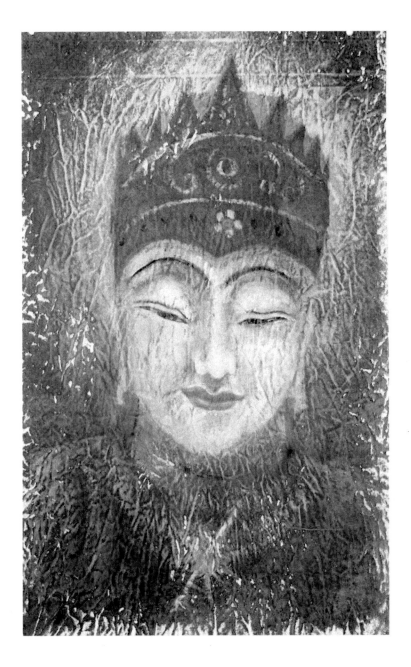

Figure 9—Thai Goddess, a painting by Lola Jones

OK, When Will I Be Enlightened?

FOCUS ON WHAT you want more of. Focus on the good things that have already happened. Focus on the fact that your Large Self is already "there," and that it calls to you constantly, and doesn't judge how long it takes or if you stray. Experience the perfection that already is.

As the Divine Openings unfold for you, you might experience increased bliss, love, laughter or any emotion. You might have improvements in work or money, attitude shifts, a breakthrough in a relationship, increased or decreased energy (temporarily), sleep changes, quieter mind (or temporarily busier mind.) You might notice tingling, physical sensations, physical detox, new inspirations, boredom, or temporary emptiness.

The best news, in any case, is there's nothing to do or work on—just be. You see, when you did clearing or "healing work" habitually, it just created more of what you were looking for. If you "work on" and focus on what's "wrong" now, you'll create more of it. Now I hope you're not creating more. It's moving and rising spontaneously, as energy is supposed to move. Your Divine Intelligence orchestrates it. Hard work is over. You can let go of the old paradigm of working on yourself now.

Appreciation will smooth your progress. Say, "Thank you for moving this old energy and feeling upward. Thank you for breaking down the old, so there's room for the new to come in." "I appreciate that what's left my life needed to go. Now what's next?"

The more you focus on what is not here, the more you delay it. The more you stress about your enlightenment, the slower it comes. Relax and enjoy the ride, and better things just come to you. Above all, it's all about joy. There's really nowhere to get *to*.

Start focusing more on how you feel right now, and less on the big outcomes.

This is not about healing, fixing, clearing or cleansing. It is simply returning to alignment with who you really are. It can be very gentle. Release any belief in growing by struggle and pain.

In general, this massive realignment process goes like this: you receive a Divine Opening and directly experience the Divine in you. Then it begins to work on you from the inside out. The pure positive bliss energy you feel also stirs up, activates, and moves many slow and dense energies/emotions/habits/resistances that are clogging the pipes. You may feel it as it moves up the scale—you may not. Then love and joy can flow through the pipes better than ever. You may go up and down for a while, and then you stabilize at a higher level. The higher level soon feels "normal" to you. Then you go higher in another cycle, and stabilize there. Increasingly you feel joy even when there's no "reason" to, or love where there was none. Eventually, nothing can get you down for long.

The farther into Divine Openings you go, the more you'll turn inward for support and communion directly with the Divine. In the early stages, though, don't hesitate to ask for support. It may feel like you're unhooking from the matrix, seeing behind the curtain, as you remember who you really are. The territory is unfamiliar, and it puts us all outside our comfort zones, but the help is there within and without. Increasingly, we can relax and let the Flow of Life show us where to go and how to get there. The "softer" we are and the more we let go, the easier it is.

I had imagined awakening would be some ethereal state where mystical visions appeared, and all my challenges stopped. There are fewer challenges. Challenges still occur, but there is more ease, and even relish, in handling them. It's a creative game. We came here to have a variety of experiences and contrasts. The contrasts are less extreme, but they are still there. They help us know even more clearly what we want. Eating the "fruit of the tree of the knowledge of good and evil" represents to me the birth of rational thinking, polarities and contrasts, and the Free Will choice to choose between the contrasts. In any given moment we can either align with The Divine in us or choose struggle. The choice is ours, but it's never final. You can re-choose.

Life has indeed become magical and full of synchronicity and ease, yet I, and others in this process, find it subtle most of the time. It's more like a steady stream of "all is well," a smooth unfolding of daily life that hums along without drama, punctuated with joy and occasional bursts of causeless bliss. Human neurology is not yet evolved to handle the extreme voltage of pure Divine Bliss all the time. It ebbs and flows. Surf it!

I promise you this—it will still feel horrible to slip down into the lower vibrations. It is supposed to! When you're not aligned with your Large Self, it is supposed to feel bad so you'll go back up. Dropping just a bit might even feel as bad as being at the bottom used to feel.

During my twenty-one days of silence, my Honeymoon With The Divine, I asked for a love like I'd never had—the compatible, co-creative, and passionate partnership I'd always wanted. Within a month of returning home, I met a lovely man so easily, so naturally, and it developed so smoothly and quickly that I marveled only upon looking back. I had thought fireworks would flare and trumpets would sound, but there was only the sound of our laughter, and a quiet peaceful flow of sweet casual experiences that seemed so inexplicably natural that I decided, "I think I'll keep doing this." It sure takes the pressure off both people to enjoy the moment and put aside the judgments of what it is supposed to be or where it's going. The voice inside had simple advice, "Enjoy!" That relationship was so much fun, and in some ways better than any before it, yet it was not forever. I enjoyed every minute of it and then let it go two years later when it was no longer a vibrational match. Some relationships have expiration dates, and there's nothing wrong with it.

In this new drama-free life, change is more easily accepted, incidents aren't traumatic, or they don't stick. The right people and things always appear at the right time, close on the heels of the need, or often even slightly before the need, in a way that serves everyone involved.

Within two years I went from no income to being prosperous. More important, I'm "independently happy"—independent of outer conditions. Anything I need comes. There's been steady growth in Divine Openings each year, and I'm happy it wasn't faster so I didn't get overwhelmed and overworked. If anything, I'm still holding back a bit on growth to maintain balance. I'm not impatient nor particularly ambitious—I do all this out of a natural enjoyment of the unfolding. Notoriety grows simply because I've helped a lot of people and they tell a lot of people.

Problems are fewer and fewer, and life isn't about problems anymore. Health has improved (I had forgotten about those health issues until just now. See how valuable it is to take note of the progress?) Energy has increased. It's a steady, upward path. The worries of past years are gone, and the occasional flicker of doubt quickly fades, either by itself, by diving into it for a few minutes, or by deliberately raising my altitude.

The mind still loves to make up scary stories. Even when you're free the mind might still say you're not. That's what that wrong-seeking missile of a mind does. I just don't believe everything I think anymore! I am keenly guided by the voice of my Large Self that sounds like me, only smarter. It's not flashy or mystical but it is constant if I stay up there where I can hear it. *The voice of God doesn't go away, but sometimes we do!* We can always return to it.

It is not necessarily a flashy thing, although it can be. Lightning never flashed and angels never sang for me, but one day it was clear that something had clicked in. "I've got it." I know my power. I know from my Large Self perspective that all is well. And so it is.

Enlightenment is just being in the Flow of Life.

It Will Become Normal

THIS FANTASTIC WAY of life was eventually accepted as "the way it is supposed to be." Clients' amazing experiences have become commonplace. I still love to marvel at them, though.

"Ah," I thought, "so this is the return to the Garden, the restoration of innocence, Heaven on Earth." Then that brought tears to my eyes, remembering that sixteen years ago I set the intention to create Heaven on Earth—I was nowhere near it, and didn't have the slightest clue how to do it, or even an inkling of what it would be like. How many times I despaired it would never happen. Only a few years before Divine Openings had I learned to raise my altitude easily and consistently—then Divine Openings continued to raise it until it was un-crashable. But this stage is only the beginning. Once we get to a high cruising altitude, the journey really gets exciting.

Sometimes I set a destination and go there, but often Life surprises me: this this book being read in over eighty countries, having a worldwide website, photographing covers for a holistic magazine, writing articles for it every month, writing a theme song for a film, writing, singing, and recording my own original music, all without striving. I'm sure the lack of attachment actually helped—things go great in our absence.

You become accustomed to each high you reach until it becomes quite normal for you, even a plateau of sorts. Then you reach for another plateau, thrill in it, and then it becomes normal. The universe expands as you expand. Seeking is no longer attractive nor needed.

Miracles are normal when you're in the flow of life—when they're not happening, that is not normal. Deep appreciation brings even more of it, so stop and rave often.

Waves of ecstasy might wash through your body during mundane activities. One day my truck wouldn't start, and there was absolutely no dip in my mood, only a tiny sense of inconvenience as I decided what to do, made a plan, and carried it out. The next day as I rode with the tow truck driver to the repair place I had chosen, I suddenly began to experience an almost orgasmic full body ecstasy for absolutely no reason. It was inexplicable by all logical standards. My truck was broken, I knew it was going to cost me time and money, and there I was in bliss, talking with the driver, enjoying a raging, passionately physical sense of being alive—life force flowing through my body, lighting up every cell.

I want to relate a rather mundane sequence of events that followed that magical experience. You might think God has better things to do than take care of our ordinary needs, but throughout the next month, I was reminded that The Indweller knows our every want. There was something being lined up for me that was better than anything I had anticipated.

Once the mechanic checked the truck, I got some unwelcome news—the warranty did not cover that particular issue, and the bill was for hundreds of dollars I had planned to use for something more fun. I used to call that "bad news," but now, without putting on any act at all, I'm pretty clear that there isn't any such thing. These days, even as I hear the "bad news," I think something like, "Well, that was unexpected... hmmm." I did have a momentary dip, but within an hour I had rebounded and determined to simply let in more money fast, which happened in the next week. The choice was simple: feel bad, point the nose of the plane downward, and create more unpleasant and costly incidents, or decide to raise my vibration, feel good, and point the nose of the plane upward, and change trajectory. That's an easy decision, isn't it? It worked, and any upset faded within hours. That's my mantra now: "Is pointing the nose down, no matter how justified I might be, worth it? Is it going to help create what I want?"

Days later, I decided it was time to purchase a new truck but quickly found that the trade-in value of my old truck was far less than I had thought. I'd have to sell it myself—and that wasn't something I wanted to take the time to do. I was definitely ready for a change, a fresh set of wheels that matched my new vibration. I simply shrugged, stayed focused on what I wanted, and walked out thinking, "Oh well, wonder what will happen to solve this?" Within hours a friend offered to buy the truck for what I owed, and was delighted at the price. I sold it to him, and walked back into the dealership ready to buy my new truck within two days. That solutions would flow in so quickly had already stopped surprising me.

In another surprise twist, the truck I had wanted was already sold. Again, not what I expected. I was immediately sure it was for the best, and sure enough, I found out I had been spared a mistake. The salesman had been wrong about the towing capacity, and it would not have pulled my horse trailer well. I proceeded to shop for another two weeks, walking car lots, comparing gas mileage and towing capacity stats, dodging salespeople's manipulations. I kept changing my mind, thinking, "Should I get a car, or a truck that will pull my horse trailer? Or get both?" I went back and forth, got myself confused, became too mental and analytical about it, and lost the flow, all uncharacteristic for me. I usually follow inner guidance rather than putting that much effort-full thought into things. One day I was out in the hundred-degree heat at noon walking a car lot, and feeling light-headed, I said to myself, "I'm working way too hard at this. This is so unlike my normal life these days to work this hard at anything, but it's especially weird to get no result. I need to get clear on what I want. I'll go home and relax." I went home and rested, going to bed early from the heat exhaustion. My love at the time bought a truck, which opened up new possibilities for pulling the trailer without me having a truck.

The new day dawned with a fresh new feeling, and the next night I spontaneously decided to stop off at a car lot just after closing, on my way home, and walked among the cars in a light carefree mood, caressed by a cool breeze. My gaze fell upon a deep metallic red convertible. My heart leaped for joy. It felt good. Suddenly, it was clear—the vehicles I'd been telling myself I should get were boring, and that was the reason I had not been able to make up my mind. In my heart of hearts I didn't really like any of them! This car *felt* good.

From out of a closed showroom, a salesman appeared, and I drove the car, thrilling at the fresh air and the open sky. I had wanted one of these convertibles, this exact model, for years, but had always thought I must have a truck, due to the horses. The salesman said the car had just come in yesterday. The reason I hadn't found it earlier was it wasn't there yet, and I was stuck on the truck idea. All my focused "working" had kept me from seeing something different than I had expected. I use this mundane example of a car, but how often do we "miss seeing it" in business, in relationship, in other areas of life?

I laugh as I think of this sequence of events—a few days in the life of a person awakening. Literally "lightening up" on the search and releasing the tension around it had loosened me up so I'd relax and have fun; so I'd once again live in the moment and be happy even before the solution occurred. You'll begin to get happy before the solution occurs, which allows you to let it in.

The moment is all there ever is, after all, and straining forward into some future moment, especially with tension, is a recipe for unhappiness in this moment. It's all about joy after all. Relaxing opened me up to be guided, and The Divine was able to show me what I really wanted.

But it wasn't the car that made me happy, it was relaxing and letting go that made me happy. Becoming happy allowed me to find the car; the car was just a byproduct of the happiness, a small material expression of that energy.

The car story also illustrates that The Divine cares about every detail of our lives, just like a best friend does. Really, cars are quite trivial in my world; I don't care what people think about what I drive or what status it confers. It just has to feel good *to me*. Feeling good is such an important indicator to me—when something feels that good I know I'm on track. The Presence wanted me to feel good and have fun when I'm driving my car—wanted me to have something that I had not let myself have for many years. Our Large Self doesn't judge what we want; it just delivers it. A friend joked, "When you go around all the time with your crown chakra open, you want a car that matches." Driving along on a cool evening, I look up at the starry sky, and appreciate my Large Self. Appreciation is the single best way to elevate your joy instantly.

At times, day to day, it may seem not much is changing, but you'll look back six months, and see much has changed. Now, just by setting *simple intentions*, forces are set in motion that shift things *for you*. Intention becomes your major tool after emotional mastery is achieved and suffering has ended. Changes in your life might be subtle or dramatic, but it doesn't matter—you're moving, and movement feels good. My work shifted from local private sessions and classes to worldwide phone sessions and mostly online courses in just a few months' time, all from a steady, clear, calm intention. That clarity and calm came from mastery of mind and emotions, guided by the Instrument Panel. Power of intention increases with attention to it. Here's a quote from my original song *Watch Where You Point That Thing* on the music collection of the same name.

Your mind is a powerful instrument.

Watch where you point that thing.

Expanding The Universe

LOOK AT ALL the things you think you need to do, be, and have—from a fine home, to education, to achieving enlightenment, to being in love, to serving others. You want all that because you think you will be happier by being, doing, or having it. See if you can think of one single thing you want that doesn't hold the promise of making you feel better—better about yourself, your loved ones, or the condition of humanity. So, here's the secret: get happy now, before you get the job or the mate, before you are enlightened, before you become who you want to be, before all wars end, before politicians tell the truth, before your mother changes, before you get rich and skinny. Then you have what you really wanted in the first place—and you have it right NOW.

The secret to happiness is to savor the waiting between the time you decide what you want and the day it arrives on the physical plane. You desire it, your Large Self creates it on the spot, indeed "becomes it," and starts the party. Your job is to let go, relax, release tension and resistance, and get your altitude up, so you're vibrating in alignment with your Large Self about it. You get yourself to the party, and you're the last key piece. Then the party appears on the physical plane.

You will always and forever be in that gap between the thought creation of the next creation you desire and the physical arrival of it, because as each dream is fulfilled, you will dream another one immediately. That is your creative nature. Get used to being "on the way to _____."

"Wanting" keeps life flowing through you. You'll either savor the waiting and be happy now, even though the next dream is not yet here, or you will always be suffering because the next dream is not yet here. Which one speeds up the arrival of your desires and which one slows them down?

Savor the waiting. Enjoy the journey. That journey turns out to be your life.

At a more advanced stage, you'll notice that the biggest thrill isn't the physical manifestation of something; the biggest thrill comes in that moment (now!) that your spirits begin to soar about it as it forms in the non-physical. You birth an intention, and you feel the Universe expanding with your creation, *as it is being created.* As you with your now heightened senses feel the energy of it lining up, you hop on that wave of your creation like a surfer, and you surf the pure energy of it while it's still in the non-physical. That non-physical swelling is as pleasurable as the physical outcome, much as a pregnant woman loves her baby before she ever sees it. The Universe enjoys the expansion you created whether you let it into your personal physical world or not, but of course you're letting it in now. Are you beginning to really get who and what you are?

You expand the Universe by creating what you want.

When your heart leaps, your soul sings, and life looks brighter—in that moment you're happy whether that manifestation ever shows up or not. Paradoxically, that's when the manifestation you so long wanted can most easily come—the job, the car, the lover, the bliss, or the enlightenment. It will seem matter of fact to you by the time it comes. "Why, of course it's here, I've been surfing on the wave of it. I didn't have to wait for it to get happy. *I took the shortcut* to happiness."

Feeling good has become such a strong habit that family dramas, even my father's life-threatening illnesses, don't sink me. Small dips, perhaps. Usually not even that. I am now like a boat that bobs to the surface no matter how many waves crash over my boat. I've been known to enjoy the rocking. This is contagious and it has buoyed up my friends and family many times in the face of serious difficulties. By being who you are, and creating the feelings and manifestations you create, you add to the Universe, which expands it. Your happiness is felt, as a tangible atmosphere, like weather, across the Universe. Really.

I'm not floating above it all, nor jaded or detached. Far from it. I am solidly grounded in my body sensations and emotions, and life is more intensely felt than ever—I just feel higher vibrations more often, and stay in the lower vibrations less. The norm is a smooth hum. I still have frequent, intense surprise attacks of sweet wonder and awe, tears stream down my face from the sweetness of a simple hug, every cell in my body feeling as if it could burst from the fullness. And that comes and goes like all feelings and experiences do. There is no way to hold onto it. Life moves. Energy wants to move. Let it move.

If Your Bliss Seems To Fade

Some people say after a few months or a year, "My high has worn off." But when I ask them to look at it, they see that they are higher, overall, than they used to be. It's now their normal state, but the initial newness and thrill is now taken for granted. And now their Large Self is calling them higher. They feel the newly opened gap between where they are now and the next level. It is true that seeking can be over with Divine Openings, but the journey of joy and expansion is endless.

This true story says it quite entertainingly. A friend took a course from me years ago, before Divine Openings. She was on food stamps, lived in a tiny rental cottage, and was depressed. After the course, she was renewed, and soon started a company that became successful worldwide.

Then she came to a Divine Openings event years later and said she was stuck. She said, "I'm right back where I was ten years ago before I took your other course! I'm single and in debt, and I'm not happy about it." I looked around the room and everyone was buying that story. I laughed and said, "Darlin', that is what the mind does to you. I beg to differ with this dire assessment. I know a bit about your life. You are vastly beyond where you were ten years ago. You are not on food stamps. You have a successful company. You own a home and horses. You travel constantly. You were just on Oprah. You got used to your new success level and now you want more. You are merely on a plateau, not letting yourself leap off and fly. You're a creative being. You want to stretch your wings further and fly higher. You came to the right place— again!"

She grinned sheepishly, then laughed. Our wrong-seeking-missile-mind can take the small-self perspective and tell the worst possible story about *any situation*. It ignores all the good and goes straight for what is wrong. It discounts our progress and pounces on what hasn't happened yet.

Experience is relative. When you fall in love with someone new, it's a rush of new feelings and sensations. Then as you are together longer, you may actually love them more, but the thrilling before-and-after contrast isn't there anymore. Humans feel contrast more than sameness, and that feeling becomes "normal" to you. The relationship deepens and the love is actually stronger and more real. Divine Openings is like that. You can tend to it and nurture it, and keep it fresh and alive and growing by raving every day about how great it is. Or you can focus on the problems, complain that the thrill is gone, and it could indeed soon be gone.

With Divine Openings, it's as if you've met and fallen in love with your Large Self, the larger part of you. It's a huge contrast from where you were, so the thrill is huge when you first feel it. It's the ultimate love affair. But you will become used to this new relationship, and even though it's always deepening, it will just feel normal. If you complain about the lack of excitement, you create more lack of it. If you constantly rave about what you have, you create more of it.

If you won the lottery, you'd jump up and down and scream, "I'm rich, I'm RICH!" But in a year you wouldn't still be doing that. Hopefully you'd appreciate it, but you would be used to it, calmer about it. You'd even begin to take it for granted. And you'd soon want more in your life.

Enlightenment cannot and will not freeze your bliss into a static thing that stays the same for ever after. That would be impossible. Energy wants to move, and life is change; your Large Self wants you to expand and grow. Use your Free Will to create new joys and fresh highs rather than expecting the old ones to stay. You're happiest when you fly ever upward on the fresh thermals of your own heart's desires no matter how modest or grand they are. It's all relative. If you are one whose desires are big, whose thermals are fast and high, you will need to keep up a brisk pace of evolution to keep up with your dreams and stay fulfilled. If you've always been content with a modest life, modest movement will keep you happy. When you cling to what was good yesterday and don't allow yourself to go to the next level, you won't feel good. When it's time to release resistance and move—let go of the old, no matter how great it has been, and go for more!

If your bliss has faded, you're holding yourself back. It's supposed to feel bad, just like the red light on your car's Instrument Panel is supposed to tell you your emergency brake is on. It's supposed to feel bad to want something and not let yourself have it. It's supposed to feel bad when your Large Self is calling you to the party, and you're not letting yourself go. Appreciate the valuable information. Get yourself to the party. Get a life. Or an expanded life.

Each Divine Opening you receive accelerates the energy, power, and momentum in your life. If you get revved up or edgy, but your life is not moving, stop receiving the Divine Openings and focus instead on relaxing, letting go, and *releasing resistance*. If you keep pushing harder on the accelerator to go faster, but also have your foot on the brake (resistance), you'll burn up your car. Blocking yourself isn't good for you and it's supposed to feel bad. Life mirrors it to you in the form of accidents, unwanted events, emotional stress, disease, or pain in your body.

"Divine Mother hugs" are calming, soothing, and resistance-releasing rather than accelerating. We give them in sessions, at live events, and on page 110 of this book. The audio called *Soothe Yourself* trains you how to do just that for yourself (see our site).

Resistance feels bad. Letting go feels good.
Your Instrument Panel works!

What To Do If:

1. **The small self grabs the controls**, you get hung up in small-self concerns, being right, working too hard, or anything low on the emotional scale. Your Instrument Panel will read a lower altitude, and it's supposed to feel bad, so you'll notice! Check who's driving, and tip the nose up. Use the *Thirty Ways To Raise Your Altitude* at the end of the book.

2. **You are not consciously creating your life.** When you choose your thoughts and feelings you can keep your altitude up consistently. If you don't choose, it's too easy to go on autopilot and let circumstances, other people, or the outer world lower your altitude. Choose! Choose is alignment with your Large Self. Then you don't have to specify the details of what you want; let it come in the perfect form for you. Co-creation is a two-way street. Sometimes you deliberately decide what you want, sometimes you put it on the God List and let go.

3. **You let outside forces influence you** and bring you down. Hold your own center. Focus inward, not outward. Stop watching TV and reading bad news. All is well within. There is an un-shakable peace there, as at the eye of the hurricane, where your Large Self always lives.

4. **An emotion wants to move, and you resist.** The emotion or the resistance may be unconscious. You don't have to go digging for the problem. Just look at your life. There will be clues. Example: People are being combative with you. Look at your life and notice any grudge you've been holding against someone, or negative thoughts about something. That's attracting aggression! That is your cue to let it go. Or suddenly, you'll see a belief that is holding you back. Relax, tip the nose up, and what you need to know comes to you.

5. **You are holding back** from something your heart wants, or from being who you really are. Life is calling you to the party and you're not letting yourself go. You know it's time for a new job, vacation, next level relationship, to write your book, perform your music, or come out of the closet, but you may have very logical reasons *(excuses!)* why you can't: "I have responsibilities, it won't work, can't afford it, can't face it, I owe it to (someone) to stay here." Move! Go! You'll feel great again once you get to the party. Let go and let The Divine do the heavy lifting.

6. **You have tipped the nose of your plane down.** You are focusing on what's wrong in your life, in the world, or on what isn't here yet. That tips the nose downward. Instead, focus passionately and rave about what *is* right, what *is* here and what you *are* grateful for. You create your world out of thin air, out of nothing, from the Fertile Void. What feelings and experiences are you generating with your focus? What world are you creating? Focus on what you want, which will flow the energy in an upward direction, and tip the nose up. Soothe yourself now.

7. **Things aren't going well, yet you're unaware of your resistance.** Set an intention. Give it over to The Divine. Let it be shown to you! You don't need to analyze it or do anything.

Check your Instrument Panel. Where are you? When you're in the lower half of it, there is resistance involved. Don't go digging for dirt; that's not necessary or productive. Observe your life. Feel and flow. Let go, ask The Divine to do the heavy lifting, and you will go higher than before.

If you get stuck in a blind spot, get help from a Divine Openings Giver. Your life is too important to let anything get you down.

Nothing is more important your vibration. It creates your reality.

More Ways To Realign With Your Large Self and Reclaim Your Happiness

1. Rave and appreciate. This is the most powerful thing you can ever do.

2. Soothe yourself. Talk to yourself like you would talk to a friend or child. Chat with The Presence. Tell yourself soothing stories. If you can't sleep, don't resist or make it wrong. Lie there and soothe yourself, and you'll arise refreshed even if you don't sleep.

3. Accept where you are. Where you are is where you are, and where else could you be? Experience where you are fully. Give it over to The Divine. It will shift faster without resistance or judgment. Deep within you, all is well *right now.* Go within and feel it for yourself.

4. Accept that your Large Self is always ahead of you. Put all the things you want on the God List and let them go. Enjoy the journey to the party. Savor each step. Soothe yourself with, "I'll get there. And then I'll want more. Enjoy now…. now…. and now."

5. Have a "Date with The Divine" and renew your romance with your Large Self. Go into the silence alone for a day without television, radio, email, phones or books. Speak to no one, and put all your focus on The Presence within. Talk only to The Presence and deepen your relationship. Talk, chat, laugh, cry, share, and appreciate. Nothing compares with that deep, sweet communion.

6. Move to uplifting music. Physical movement and play blasts you upward in vibration. *Watch Where You Point That Thing* comes with a movement video link that's all about joy.

7. Remember who you are. You are a Divine being in a physical body. You chose to come here and experience contrasts, choose among choices, and co-create with The Creator.

8. Meditate regularly, even if for only ten minutes. It focuses you on what is real—the inner you, your Larger Self, the silence. Divine Openings has opened up your ability to meditate more deeply than ever before. Don't do it to "work on yourself" but to feel good. Meditate for pleasure.

9. Breathe for pleasure. Breathe in and out gently and naturally as you focus on your breath. Let your spine undulate with the breath. Relax. Don't work. Think soft. Emotions might arise and move. If they do, relish them. Be with them until they move up. Sometimes you can get to bliss. If you're over-revved or can't sleep this is a fabulous thing to do. Enjoy!

You'll begin to feel peace or bliss again as soon as you take one step, tip the nose up slightly, and deliberately soar upward. Bliss is the natural result of soaring on the flow of Life. The moment your energy stops flowing freely, or even slows down, you feel less good. There's a longer list of easy practices at the end of the book. Play at it—don't work!

Happiness is your natural state. Releasing resistance returns you to it.

Whether a heart's desire is thwarted, or your nose has drifted downward, your bliss will fade as the vibration drops and gets denser! Your Large Self is always moving and expanding, flying along on the current of *your desires*. It's not resisting at all. It's already at the party. Your party. Not allowing yourself to go too will feel bad, and it's supposed to.

You must expand and flow with the current of Life in order to feel good again. That means feeling it all, wherever you are on the Instrument Panel. That means following your heart, whatever it wants. That means disregarding your mind, it's limits, and whoever or whatever says you can't.

You must let go to the flow. It might mean moving to Denmark, but it might be as simple as doing something mundane in your own back yard that makes your heart sing. It doesn't have to be any big deal. When I want to go thrift store shopping, I go. It relaxes me, and for some odd reason, makes my heart soar. I can afford brand new clothes, but that doesn't give me the same zing. Go figure. I often visualize what I want to find there, and there's a big sense of adventure and wonder at where I'll find it, and how soon. Sometimes it's the same day. The important thing is to do it simply because I feel like doing it. You must buck the consensus reality, and venture outside it.

Recently I had reached another plateau and was feeling rather normal and mundane instead of blissful, though other people would say to me, "You're so peaceful," or "I get high being around you" (it's all relative.) But we must each stay up with our own heart desires; someone else's norm may not be enough for you or me. Since the natural urge of living beings is to expand and find ever greater levels of release and joy, I began to want more—and apparently I was holding back, because I could feel resistance in my body, especially tension in my neck!

Your Instrument Panel always tells you when it's time to expand. First you'll notice a subtle nudge from your Large Self—a thought or a desire. If you ignore that, you'll feel your emotions slide down the Altimeter. If you ignore your emotions, it escalates, and you'll start to experience physical symptoms like tension or stiffness or pain. If you ignore the subtle physical signals, illness could occur. It's a progressive system where your Instrument Panel flashes increasingly brighter warning lights and blares louder buzzers to tell you you're resisting.

While teaching a Divine Openings Course years ago, it became clear: I realized that like some of the students that day, I was still buying into the consensus reality that "work is hard" and "money is hard," thought forms that are completely pervasive in our scarcity-riddled world. I had begun to pick up a little stress, which is just information, a signal to *move, expand, let go*!

I decided (*intention* is all it takes at this stage) to create even more ease for myself. Each time we *intend* new avenues open up, and new inspirations are magnetized to help us. In the seminar we all dived into the vibration that lies at the heart of the feeling that work is hard and money is scarce. It rose in vibration, and I soon found myself tickled to the point of giggling to myself at that absurd old notion. A new lightness came over me.

Releasing resistance by fully feeling through it restored my high. Then that momentum brought even more progress. In this new consciousness, the next day a new chain of events began unfolding effortlessly. First I got depressed! Of course, my mind protested, "This isn't progress! I'm going backwards. I don't get depressed anymore. Shouldn't this enlightenment stuff make me immune from this?" But my Large Self gave me a quiet soothing feeling, assurance that this was perfect and if I didn't resist it would pass quickly. Resistance to feeling creates suffering.

I sat on the porch on a perfect day and dived into the vibration that felt like "depression," sensing that this was very old energy. I began to feel lighter and lighter and soon lost interest in the exercise, which is usually your cue that you are done with it. I brought my laptop out to write, and soon, with no effort, I felt better than I had in weeks—it was a new high.

There was a domino effect as more guidance came in—I had a very subtle and easy urge to skip the glass of wine with dinner. A glass of wine occasionally is fine, but I felt a desire to get even more sparkling clear for a week or so, and I wanted to maximize this new rise in altitude.

For many, alcohol gives that permission to feel extra good, as if somehow it's "not your doing." But you can feel good without any reason, and it's OK! I have a drink occasionally, but I love natural highs, and I'm so accustomed to being up there that the substances and activities many people use to get high actually are a downward move for me. It's all relative.

The result of following this inwardly guided trail of mundane changes was that more money began to flow in with less work. I didn't analyze. I just felt and followed.

Notice that I don't often use euphemisms like abundance and prosperity. Many spiritual people use those fluffy words because they have judgments about money and can't bring themselves to say "I want money." So, check yourself. Can you say, "I want cash"? Abundance and prosperity aren't accepted as legal tender and won't pay for groceries or rent. Money will.

The big message is to follow your urges and pay attention to how you feel. All else will come.

Feel and follow.

Do Things Just Because They Feel Good

THE UPWARD MOMENTUM continued, and I soon felt a whole new spontaneous level of permission to feel good. Most of us have some cultural taboos that we don't know we have. There are "unquestioned assumptions," things we bought into without questioning them because everyone else believed it, and then it became part of the background of life, like the air you never notice you're breathing. Growing up, we pick up from the culture and the adults around us that we shouldn't feel *too* good, be too boisterous, enjoy our body or sex too much, or be "too greedy." We should work hard and not be "lazy" or decadent. We've been told desire is bad.

Desire for expansion, for opening, and for "more" is what drives the universe. It doesn't have to be profound or "for a lofty purpose." It can be just because your wanting it moves delightfully delicious energy through you, and that movement expands the universe. Your fulfilling your desires forwards life in the universe. Feeds it. Expands it. Your joy sends out a ripple that lights up the universe. You're that valuable. Your peace and joy are that important.

Desire that feels like craving things you think you can't have hurts you. That kind of desire feels bad. Craving for a partner, or money or success while feeling a gnawing lack of that in your gut— that hurts, and tips the nose down.

If you want to make a difference in the world, be joyful. It makes you a broadcast tower radiating a vibrational message of love, joy, and power.

Somehow, that Puritan ethic had snuck in there and put some limits on my pleasure, but suddenly I saw it and popped out of it. Again, totally spontaneously, I began to do new things just because they felt good; I would lie in bed in the mornings, at nap time, or at bedtime, and just luxuriate in the softness of the sheets, enjoy the sensations on the skin, smile at the many things there are to appreciate about a simple bed. I'd snuggle my cheek on the pillow, and stretch out catlike in languorous delight at the sound of the wind in the trees. I took a long hot bath with candles. I walked on my land, not for exercise this time, but for pleasure. Profound bliss came over me. Ahh, I had missed that feeling. It was like coming home. We love the game of getting lost and coming home as much as babies love peek-a-boo.

The greatest bliss always occurs at the point of a new energetic expansion.

On New Year's Eve, once again, I woke feeling rather flat. I'd given myself some time off of teaching and counseling; I had slept late, and I couldn't quite get my motor started. This was odd. I usually wake ready to go, go, go, powered by Source Energy. I even know how to generate energies when there aren't any (we do create it all.) .

But that day, after a great breakfast of pancakes and sausage, I got an inspiration to do a project I'd wanted to do for years. I love puttering around the ranch and making things more functional and beautiful. The Fort Worth cowgirl in me loves building fences, fixing up the barn, and organizing things so they work better. For five years I had I wanted a door out the back of the feed room straight out to the barn so that when it's rainy and cold I could feed the horses without getting wet. With a friend who loves doing ranch chores, we started on it, and then he needed some time to just do it without me looking over his shoulder.

So I did one of my other favorite things. I got on my John Deere garden-tractor-riding-mower and mowed giant spirals in the tall yellow grass in the front pasture. The folks in the upcoming Five-Day Silent Retreat could walk this labyrinth while they integrated their special Divine Openings. Then I kept going and mowed about three more acres just for fun. I'm like a kid when I ride the mower. It's like riding a go-cart, and watching the land become manicured and beautiful gives me a lot of satisfaction. Add that to seeing the new door in the feed room almost complete, and I cannot describe to you the thrill I felt as the sun went down. It was ecstatic. I don't know why it feels so good to do those things, and I don't care. It doesn't matter why something feels good to you. It doesn't need to have a point, it doesn't even have to be productive, and no one else needs to understand it. Just do it. You're adding to the joy in the universe.

You may feel like you have "too much work to do" to allow yourself to do things that are not income producing or responsible. But you must do the things your heart wants to do; those things are literally food for your soul, and if you starve your soul, how can you be productive? You have no idea how much those "useless" things fuel your income-producing efforts. Since there is no deadline saying you have to do them, your weeks can continue to fly by without ever doing them—unless you give yourself permission now.

What is it for you? Painting a picture, gardening, having coffee with a friend, teaching the dog tricks, or playing with kids? It doesn't have to be profound. Do what you feel called to do in each moment, no matter how trivial it seems. Your Large Self leads you in mysterious ways.

That very night after the fun ranch projects were done, my energy and passion skyrocketed. I had some big inspirations that led to "productive action" in my work, and they were fun ideas to carry out—outside the box ideas. I felt renewed and enthusiastic about going to a New Year's Eve party, where before I was ambivalent about whether to go out, and I met lots of interesting new people and had a great time. I met a woman who could help me with some technical challenges. Doing those simple heart's desires led me on a productive, upward path.

Let go of "shoulds" and judgments about being a realistic, responsible adult, and instead, go with your heart's desires at least once a day—if not five or six times. You'll be amazed at what happens in other areas of your life when you step into that flow. When people say they're working harder to make their business grow, I'll grin and say, "Take a vacation. Things will go great in your absence."

As I followed my feelings further, I realized I really wanted to stop doing so many private sessions and do courses instead. I'm not a "routine" person. I was tired of teaching the same things over and over, one-to-one. Within a month I began doing mostly courses. Then rapidly I got clear that online classes would work, and three people who knew how to set that up had already showed up in my life and suggested ways to do it. Soon I was helping ten times more people in one fifth of the time it used to take. Magic.

Do things that feel good to you.

ACTIVITY: List some things you could do this week, just to feel good!

1.
2.
3.
4.
5.
6.
7.
8.
9.
10.

Now, what are you waiting for? Do them!

Dream Intentions

DREAM INTENTIONS (I used to call them dream assignments) are one of my favorite ways to create, since in dream state we have zero resistance. While asleep, we are fully open to our Large Self—set free from the density and limits inherent in human form. It's the least resistant we will ever be while in physical bodies. We revert to pure non-physical consciousness and rest, recharge, create, and play unfettered in the loving Presence of our Pure Divine Source.

I write down things my Large Self can take care of for me while I sleep, or just intend it as I drift off to Resistance-Free Land. After setting Dream Intentions, I let them go, breathing with a big sigh, "It's not my job. It's done." It's fun to create Dream Intentions with your partner.

It's like delegating, but delegating up. Remember the idea of *bhakti paradina*, the God who is at your service? Think of it like your own personal assistant who never sleeps, knows everything and everyone, and cheerfully works for you twenty-four hours a day, beyond time and space. Appreciate that this Larger You never sleeps, and can do anything. With Divine Openings, when you sleep, things go great in your absence. It's especially great now that life is about creating rather than just solving issues and problems—creating fun and adventure, designing your life however you want it. Do a quick check and notice which you're doing. Remember, you'll get what you expect!

You sleep better when you "give over" all your cares and concerns first. Go to sleep on a good note, and you rest better. Off-loading all your cares gives profound peace, releases resistance, and brings relief. If you're overwhelmed, make a list, give it to The Divine and let go. Inspiration will come later when you least expect it. Better yet, many things on the list just show up or get done without any effort. I like running across an old list—invariably, most of it is done—much of it without much effort from me. Or it never needed to be done. Something better came along that made it unnecessary.

"Bad" dreams with Divine Openings mean Grace is raising that lower vibration for you. There is nothing to analyze, do, or worry about. *It's not predicting anything bad.* Say soothingly to yourself, "It's being handled in my absence."

Dreams aren't just about solving problems; they're about cooking your desires and creations. I particularly like Dream Intentions when my desire is big, since my limiting thoughts and beliefs often can't fathom how it can happen. There are no limits in the non-physical, or in dreamland.

Divine timing may not agree with my timing, but if I give it over and wait, it always comes eventually, or something better happens. It's much better than wearing myself out trying to do it all myself, forcing my own timetable. So many things we think we have to do are just the mind's incessant nagging. They were never necessary, or wouldn't have worked anyway.

Remembering the dream or getting the answer" is *not important*. You may remember nothing when you wake, yet the thing you asked for shows up spontaneously in synchronistic ways in good timing. Someone gives you a lead, a person or piece of information shows up, or an inspired idea enters your mind later when you least expect it. Dream Intentions are great for anything—business, money, personal, relationship, creative, and health—desires of any kind.

Dream on it.

Just Ask, Then Let Go!

WITH ALL OF these processes and techniques, we could forget the simplest and most powerful thing of all. Letting go and letting The Divine do the heavy lifting is always the most powerful thing you can do.

Talk to The Presence and chat about what you need and want. But don't keep asking over and over. It's done. Keeping on asking contradicts it and says you don't think it's done.

The party started when you asked. Focus on how you can get out of the way, release resistance, and get yourself to the party. For the simplest and most mundane needs, for realizing your dreams, communications with loved ones, business and money, relief of physical illness, the wisest decision, the best vacation plan, for humor and fun, The Presence knows what you want, and starts the party. Get yourself to the party.

The Divine is already offering help in every moment, way before you ask, but your asking focuses *your* energy and aligns *you* with the solution. It reminds you to look for and let in the answers that are always being offered. It focuses you on getting to the party.

The most powerful thing you can ever do is give it over to The Presence, the Larger You.

How To Teach It? Live It!

SOMETIMES PEOPLE ASK how they can influence their families and co-workers to live an enlightened and happy life. With much experience behind me, my best answer is clear: live it and let them see that. Let it take as long as it takes. Your example is the best teacher, and our efforts are best spent practicing it rather than preaching it. You'll know for sure you're living it when they're getting it. You can roughly gauge your awakening by how much those around you are awakening.

And I don't mean be perfect at it. Being an example of it can mean saying, "Hey, I'm angry at you right now, so let's not talk until I have a chance to clean up my own feelings. I'm going for a walk to do just that. I'll be back. See you in a bit." Wow, what a powerful message! You're claiming your power instead of blaming them. This teaches kids to feel and be authentic, yet responsible.

In an old relationship before Divine Openings, I kept wishing the man would do more personal development with me. Instead, he would continually bust me when I wasn't walking the talk, and he seemed to delight in doing things to get me to lose control of my emotions.

At the time it was pretty frustrating, but now I see that he was not able to hear my wise words because my frequent unwise actions spoke louder. Back then I wasn't yet able to consistently live what I was teaching. I do live it now, although not always in every single moment, but I've gotten so much better at it. I manifested kinder partners by becoming kinder to myself, and raising the old vibrations that attracted unkindness before.

It's easier to teach others formally when you are doing this professionally, and they officially consent by asking you or signing up for it. That gives you permission to teach them. I don't teach informally to friends and family. I mind my own business. I might say, "Ask if you want to hear my perspective," or "Would you like input, or are you just wanting me to listen?" It doesn't help if someone doesn't want it. When you give advice someone hasn't asked for, it can even feel like an attack or a criticism.

Think about those cop shows on television where a crime is committed against one of the detective's family members, and he goes out to avenge the crime. His superior tells him he's off the case because he's too emotionally attached. He goes against orders and goes after the criminal, causing all kinds of havoc. You'll find it feels tense when you're not minding your own business.

When you're too attached, "take yourself off the case."

Our site does all the work for you if you want to share Divine Openings. There's a place on www.DivineOpenings.com to send emails to your friends to introduce them to the site. We give you a free gift for sharing. Let go of attachment to their response. You've done your good deed by offering, and that feels good in itself.

There are moments in everyday life when I realize a person cannot hear me from where they are. I must sound like I'm speaking in some foreign tongue. In those moments, when they are complaining, suffering, and nose-diving, and can't even see the possibility of a solution, I take a deep breath and say from the heart, "I hear you. It sounds tough." I stop talking, mind my own business, and walk the talk. It's their life, and pushing too hard to help is being controlling. Let others have their choices. They may surprise you and suddenly one day be open, or find another teacher they can hear better. There are different teachers for different people.

If you *are* truly called from within to teach formally, nothing will stop you from doing it. Doors will open, and it will start happening. You may choose to be initiated in the Five-Day Silent Retreat to give Divine Openings, or you can radiate that Grace from any profession. You can also do the retreat just for your own expansion and liberation.

Practice rather than preach.

Daydream For "Entertainment"

DAYDREAMS ARE FUN, and like meditation, are even more powerful than the relief from resistance you get at night, because you are consciously creating them. Exercising your focus as a conscious creator strengthens your power of intention, just as a muscle gains power from exercise.

There is no difference between a vivid daydream and reality, for the purposes of creating. Olympic athletes have used powerful visualization for years to improve their performance. Whenever you get a chance, daydream about what you want for yourself, and what you want to see in the world. That's all your Large Self sees anyway, all the time!

Daydreaming feels good because it aligns you with your Large Self. Your Large Self has already created that reality you want, and is just waiting for you to stop getting in the way and sending out resistant contradictory energy. It's waiting for you to get up to altitude with it so it can manifest in the physical. Best of all, it feels good right now!

You are not daydreaming to create something; it's already created. You were heard the first time you felt the desire, and your request was granted instantly. The party is happening in the non-physical realm right now, and it pops into the physical faster if you don't contradict and reverse it.

So often you're on the way to your desire, vibrating high about it, feeling great—then something in the outer world doesn't go like you expected, and you let your vibration go down. Now you're headed in the opposite direction of your desire. Don't let the outer world and it's happenings influence you. Operate as if your vibration is the only thing that's important—because it *is* the only thing that matters ultimately. Anything happening in the outer world is temporary.

Daydreaming relaxes you so you don't contradict your desire with resistance, doubts, and slow down the manifestation. You daydream to get yourself to the party.

Daydreaming is a powerful way to savor the waiting and get out of the way.

Visualize mainly to keep yourself happy and out of the way.

Most of what we think, feel and vibrate was programmed and conditioned into us from birth. We got trained out of our natural Grace state. Much of our thoughts, feelings and the content of our current lives are not our own conscious creation, but more a mish-mash of hand-me-down ideas, beliefs, and thoughts from our family, society, and Ancient Mind. Now we get a fresh start.

Do your daydreaming for entertainment, and you will have the most relaxation and the least possible resistance on that subject. If you tell yourself it's for fun and not serious work, you'll relax, let go, and enjoy—and guess what? That's the very attitude that gets the fastest results.

Give yourself some short daily "inner movie time." Add sights, sounds, smells, textures, dialogue and full-fledged feelings to your daydream script. Make it as real as you possibly can and stop if you lose the good feeling. Smile to yourself. Walk around in it rather than watching it. Add humorous scenes and you'll relax and release even more resistance. If you need help getting started, go test drive the car or horse, paint a picture, or cut out pictures and make a dream board that gives you the *feeling*, the vibration of what you want.

One man set his table with an extra plate *and food* for the ideal match who would soon show up in his life, and talked with her during meals. Now that is vibrating it right now. And yes, she did show up. An attorney daydreamed to lighten up before an upcoming hearing he was stressed about, and he smiled as he put humorous scenes in his movie. It worked. His hearing went smoothly. When you're relaxed, your power is freed up, and you'll perform miracles.

You're always "manifesting." You can't stop it.
You're just learning to do it deliberately rather than unconsciously.

ACTIVITY: Stop reading. Try just one minute of daydreaming right now. Pick something you'd love and dramatize it. Make it juicy.

You can use daydreaming to help enlighten the world and create peace. First, get *yourself* there.

You can do more good lying in your bed daydreaming what you want to see happening in the world than any legion of politicians, diplomats, missionaries, spiritual teachers, or soldiers can ever accomplish with action. So often, their tension and the "pushing against" actually creates more of the discord they are supposedly trying to eliminate. They get in discord within themselves. I rarely see a happy activist. Action doesn't produce results. Energy alignment produces results. Action just completes what was already done in the non-physical—but it often looks like it was the action that did it.

When this altruistic daydreaming practice feels good that tells you that you are in alignment with your Large Self. Simply lie relaxed and close your eyes. Create a daydream in which all is well, all is working out and everyone is prospering. As your power increases, you can offset thousands or even millions of people who are broadcasting negativity.

For thousands of years, a few enlightened masters at a time have balanced the negativity of the rest of humanity in this very way, since high vibration is thousands of times more powerful than low vibration. Now you can help.

Remember, the more like entertainment and the less like work it feels, the more powerful it is. If you get all serious or sad or angry about it, you're not contributing. Do it lightly and joyfully, and don't try to *make* anything happen. Try two more minutes of daydreaming right now, and make it fun!

Empty and Meaningless

ONE MORNING, some months after going through my twenty-one days of silence, I woke up and noted matter-of-factly that everything seemed pointless, and that was OK with me. Since I had been in a state of pretty constant happiness with frequent blasts of bliss since I got back, this was "interesting," but in my typical equanimity, I knew there was nothing wrong—I'd just be with it. I went efficiently about my work as if nothing was different. That's one thing that has been radically different since I began Divine Openings. Nothing stops me, and I go on with what needs to be done no matter how I feel. It's as if The Presence just moves my body. Things just perk along on a kind of super-efficient Divine autopilot. There's an invisible motor always running.

Since I didn't resist it, I got over this empty and meaningless bout in about half a day! Things move through you fast once you are willing to be with whatever is. Soon I was excited that we had come that far, that the empty and meaningless stage of enlightenment that classically used to last months or years was happening in mere hours for me and my clients.

One day soon after, a friend hit the same stage. He said he sat staring blankly at the wall for hours, and had become quiet—very odd for him! Being an action person, he normally would have either talked about his concerns, worked out, or done something to distract himself. For some time had resisted giving up the fight that was so deeply ingrained in him. My guess is that in his despair and fatigue, he gave up, a crack of least resistance appeared, and Grace took over and stopped him in his tracks.

He was in a detached state, and had little to say except, "Everything feels empty and meaningless. The worst thing is nothing even seems funny. My writing depends on humor!" He grimaced. I did catch him off guard and made him laugh by saying "Hey, what an opportunity! You could go have some empty and meaningless sex!" Then I left him alone to resume his bewildered staring at the wall. Every stage is valuable—a death of the old, and an opening to a new perception. So much of what we think is significant is not. He was soon on fire with more energy than ever, and on to a new phase of his business.

Now after years of Divine Openings, some of my biggest expansions are ushered in by a short depression or unidentifiable despair, which you can imagine is a bit scary. At first I think, "I've really lost it! Something's wrong!" But when I remember to just experience it with no resistance it can move very fast. Every single time, it turns out to be some ancient blind spot dissolving, or something I'm just now able to let go of. It's telling me "It's time to expand or let go yet again!" It's supposed to feel bad to hold yourself back or deny yourself expansion! One night I went to bed after a day of darkness of the soul, and a light being came in the night (it wasn't a dream) and offered a hand to lift me up. Then came some very soothing dreams. I woke incredibly happy the next morning. Later in the day, in a light conversation with a Divine Openings Giver, a blind spot in my life became visible and it just cleared up. Bliss erupted. That's typical.

A "dark night of the soul" is a very deep, auspicious, and blessed event that takes you higher in the end. Don't panic. You haven't "lost it." You'll come through just fine. Now, if you made it wrong, gave your power away, and turned to something or someone to "fix it" or figure out "why" it happened, that could get in the way of the natural process. Off you'd go down some detour, and back into seeking you'd go. It could go on for years with no relief no matter how hard you worked on it. If you do need help a Divine Openings Giver always leads you back inside, to yourself.

Now What?

SOMEONE GAVE ME a greeting card. One monk is opening a birthday present from another monk and as he looks into the empty box, he says, "Wow, just what I always wanted—NOTHING!" Meditate to get to nothing rather than something. Pure nothing is the essence of The Presence. All else is transitory form—mere stuff. Living "from nothing" is fresh and freeing.

We're often reluctant to let go of stuff we don't even like. When we do let go, we find out how much we defined ourselves by all that stuff. Once I helped a friend pack up his possessions to move, and he had to sort through and discard twelve years' worth of stuff. He sat on the floor, in a big pile of history, shoulders drooping. I asked him if he wanted the stuff, and he said, "No, but it still feels like a loss to let it go." I sat quietly with him and offered, "Let the feelings be. They won't last long if there's no resistance."

The body and the small self may perceive a loss. "Losing" anything, particularly letting go of a lot at once, leaves a void, and we don't like emptiness much until we get used to it.

As much as we all have wanted our life to transform, when it does, it can feel joyful . . . disconcertingly unfamiliar… joyful… confusing… empty… joyful…

When you experience way more bliss than you're used to, even that can be disconcerting. Our small self doesn't know what the heck is going on—great things are happening and it is not in control of them. It can get frightened! "What if it doesn't last?" Someone shared that the acceptance she received to her music since her first Divine Opening was "almost scary." Her body was "opening up," and she had to "try to not be afraid, listen and follow." Isn't it interesting how the small-self fears the new, even when it's what we've always wanted?

My personal experience has covered the spectrum of emotions, and I've fully experienced them all. The joy and laughter outweighed the speed bumps, and seeing things about myself I didn't like. It felt like a tornado had swept through and cleanly wiped the slate.

"Hmm, I don't think I'm in Kansas anymore," I murmured to myself. "So, where am I? Standing on a new and unfamiliar frontier. Oh, My God—that means no road map! No map? Heck, there are no *roads!*" I felt very powerful, but was still feeling my way along.

If you want to create something new and fresh, would you paint over a canvas that was layered with thick, old paint? Or would you start on a fresh, smooth, clean, primed canvas? When you want a fresh, clean state of consciousness, start with a nice, clean, blank mind. It will feel very odd at first. Savor the emptiness for a while. It won't last. Whatever you do, don't make it wrong or resist it. It's OK. (Everything is OK.) There is no rush. Let go of your old goal-oriented way of thinking and relax for a bit. There is plenty of time in eternity. Inspiration comes, and then you move. Nature abhors a vacuum. Just be selective about what you fill it with!

When the old is gone, we stand empty and free.
And then we choose to create whatever we want.

You get to create the new life and the new world you want. There is no set destiny, although you may have incarnated with some general ideas of what you wanted to experience and what your talents would be. It's your blank canvas to paint however you please. God doesn't even dictate how God will interact with you—you get to co-create that, too! Six months after my twenty-one days of silence, I once again "upgraded" my concept of God, throwing out yet another pile of concepts I realized I had picked up in India and elsewhere that were not authentic to me or outlived their value.

After experiencing some physical pain and seeing that it was resistance (it always is), I asked within, while sitting in contemplation, "What is a truer concept of God for me *now?*" Instantly, an image of me leafing through a blank book filled with handmade paper appeared in my mind. I laughed. God is a blank book. That initiated a deeper understanding that the most pure experience of The Presence is formless, experienced in the deep silence of The Void. I threw out even more second-hand images and concepts and opened wider. From deep within emerged a Presence that was virtually impossible to describe. I heard the wind outside, and it seemed to be its/our breath. How we experience The Presence evolves as we evolve. Take your sweet time.

Looking Forward

JOY IS NOT a product of something; joy is an innate quality of your Large Self that is natural and essential. It can spill out of you like a fountain when you least expect it, in situations others might find miserable—like when my truck broke down. Without the interference of the mind, there is joy in anything. It's all experience.

Joy isn't dependent on outer circumstances, finances, approval, or events; *it just is*. Your Large

Self sits in the eye of the hurricane, at peace no matter what is going on, while your small, separated self could be unhappy or in pain if things are not going right, tossed about by the winds of its own self-created storms. The small self requires things to go a certain way to be happy while your Large Self can find happiness in any situation. The small self can experience pleasure when things are going its way, but not true joy.

Once awakened, you still experience aversion to some things and attraction to others, and like some people better than others, but there is less charge and judgment in your dislike. There are simple preferences and choices. We came here to pick and choose from options and contrasts.

Emotions come and go, but there is less charge on them, less resistance to them, so they don't "stick"; they move fluidly through you, and you don't turn pain into suffering. At first, you move in and out of blissful states, but as you stabilize, you experience the higher, finer vibrations more of the time. One minute you may feel anger or powerlessness, but you're rubberized and you quickly bounce to the top of the Altimeter, which is now your genuine set point.

The mind might still be concerned with survival, and sometimes negative or fearful—but at some point you're liberated from it, able to de-clutch from it. You ignore it a lot. You realize: *You don't have to believe everything you think. Your thoughts are not You. You are not your mind or your emotions.*

The thoughts that drift in from Ancient Mind are not yours. If a thought makes no sense, ask, "Is this mine?" If not, if will evaporate. Each time someone gets that, Ancient Mind weakens.

Your brain still works once you let go to your Divine Self, in fact, far more of it works, but the parts of it that are dominant are the parts that can sustain enlightened thought. The reptilian brain at the base of the skull is soothed and less active, less dominant. The chatty parietal lobes at the sides of the skull are quieter. The more evolved frontal lobes light up and become more active, as they tune in to God-energy and produce more inspired thought.

You waste less energy on mind-chatter. Your brain works for you when you need it, and sits quietly and idle when you don't. The thoughts that do come through it are of a higher quality and more often inspired. If your mind is busy with productive thought, that's OK. You came here to engage in this world, not sit on a cloud, empty-headed *all* the time.

Your mind is more of a receptor for Divine Intelligence and Grace, serving you rather than running you. You keep it in a more empty, free-space state rather than storing up so many events, feelings, patterns, strategies and facts; you know that what you need comes to you in the moment.

As you've heard, the "brain as a storage cabinet" is an outmoded notion. In the past we thought we needed to store up experiences and create patterns of response and defense so we could use them as guidance and protection in the future, but past experience is obviously not the best guide if we want to go beyond the past. Direct knowing is available in the moment we need it. Too often, past experience just limits what is possible.

Now we're free of the past. Things are happening that have never happened before in the history of mankind, and the pace of the expansion of human consciousness is increasing daily.

Enlightenment won't necessarily bring on mystical abilities and gifts, though it can. Psychic ability, channeling, healing, and mystical visions are more accurate and potent in people of higher vibration, but don't give flashy phenonena too much reverence. Not all people who have those abilities are enlightened.

Since we love flash and tend to compare our experiences with those of others, an important thing to remember as you experience your awakening is that you don't need flashy phenomena to be fully awakened. If your heart opens and you become quietly loving and compassionate to your entire family, this is by far more valuable than any mystical gift or visions, and does as much good for the world as any famous person working with thousands of people.

My experiences have been perfect for me, and I am fully satisfied with them—I'm not seeking anything. It's all about joy. If you go speeding through the Universe seeking wild experiences without joy, it's all pointless.

Measure your wealth and enlightenment in love and joy.

You're Never "Finished"

CAN YOU IMAGINE God complaining, "Geez, when will this creation ever be done? I have worked and worked and worked on it for eons, and still it's not done! When am I ever going to be able to relax and retire?" Sounds silly, doesn't it? But that's what we do. We want it to be done, finished, perfect, over. For what? What else do we have to do with eternity?

Creation expands forever; the game is verdant, rich, multi-faceted, infinite creation. The Creator in us cannot stop creating. Energy moves through us, generating expansion, creating an exhilarating current that our Large Self rides for fun. When we learn to ride it for fun, we've mastered the game, and we get to enjoy it as much as our Large Self does. When we march through life seeking and not finding, trying to get somewhere, there is no joy, and we are out of step with our Large Self.

Sometimes people who are progressing more slowly ask me why others they read about on our website have such miraculous results so quickly. I can offer some valuable clues. The people who get free and happy the fastest:

- Let go of everything they knew from the past, and don't mix modalities.

- Stop seeking, enjoy life, and stick with Divine Openings, which points them within.

- Appreciate all feelings. Don't resist any feeling or make it wrong.

- Take everything within to The Presence instead of talking about it to other people, whether friends or therapists.

- Stop telling their old stories. Period.

- Claim responsibility for their own reality, even when they don't yet understand how they created a particular thing. They say, "I created it," in a kind, compassionate way.

- Let go of control and don't try to figure it out intellectually.

- Make a powerful decision to stop looking to the outer world for validation or clarity.

- Commit without reservation to create their own reality, and stick to that.

- Don't take score too soon. Focus only on what's working, not what isn't. Delete "failures" and don't count them.

- Practice appreciation and rave daily.

- Read this book many times, letting in more of it each time as consciousness expands.

- Stop working on themselves, but prioritize their happiness. Divine Openings help if they do need it.

- Have the intention to slow down and savor life rather than to speed through it.

Note that none of that is working on yourself!

Most people move quickly with Divine Openings, but I want you to know that some don't choose to let go so easily. One client who described herself as resistant finally realized after over two years of Divine Openings that she'd been trying every trick in the book to not have to feel deeply. She thought there must be some loophole, some way around it. And she didn't even have childhood trauma, she was simply running from messy human feelings; a perfectionist wanting life to be perfect. She then began to open up, let go, and live life, but still hadn't ventured into relationship—she was procrastinating about dating, thinking she'd have to kiss a few toads.

Three years into Divine Openings she sent me a little gift with a note saying she was embarking on a new career, and that a man in her apartment complex knocked on her door one day and asked her out, and they've been together since. It happened just that easily, sans frog kissing, and they are perfectly compatible.

One client would complain to me that her sister had gotten the full bliss of Divine Openings but she wasn't getting it. She persistently held onto the story that all her problems were her husband's fault, and nothing could sway her. It was quite comical watching this tiny irritated woman bossing her big burly, easy-going guy around, and fortunately he was infinitely patient. Finally after two years, I heard from her again. She gleefully wrote me that she had finally just let it go and claimed responsibility for her own happiness, and she and her husband were in love like teenagers again, their relationship was better than it had been in twenty years, and she finally got "the bliss."

When you stop waiting for someone else to change or fix your life, or seeking for some magic bullet that will save you from ever feeling bad again, and start living life now, you can expand forever with ease and joy. When you're willing to experience it all, there's nothing to run away from, or seek an answer to. However long your awakening takes is OK with you, because you know your enjoyment of each moment of eternity is all that ever matters. You know there is no goal except how you feel right now.

Make peace now with your ever-expanding, never-ending journey through eternity. Laugh at the old notion of ever getting somewhere, becoming perfect, or "getting it all done." You'll die with an undone to-do list, but since there is no death, it doesn't matter. You'll continue on.

You, infinite being, are never complete.

Divine Opening

THIS IS SOUL'S DANCE. Intend to do your soul's dance full out.
Gaze at this image for one minute, then close your eyes
and savor for fifteen or more minutes.

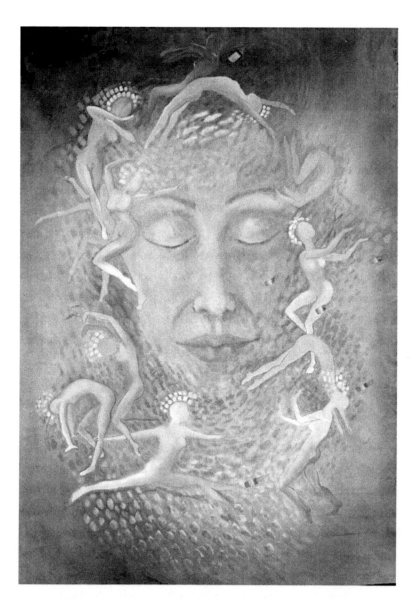

Figure 10—Soul's Dance, painting by Lola Jones.

How The Unfolding Might Go For You

MOST PEOPLE BEGIN to glimpse a new dimension of living in about a month with Divine Openings, if they're feeling, going within, and not diluting it with other stuff. Others take longer. This book, which is at Level One, usually gets people out of suffering, anxiety, and worry, and it gets most people to quiet joy and inner peace, or higher. Now you have a whole new awareness of how you're creating your reality, but most importantly, what is primary is that you know how to raise vibration and feel better. That allows you to increasingly manifest more deliberately.

If your liberation is not well underway at the end of the first reading, I invite you to read the book again, slowly. Your consciousness expands after each reading, so you'll hear and see things you would swear were not in the book before. You'll feel, let go of, and do things you resisted before. During the second reading, one woman realized she'd merely taken it in at the intellectual level on the first reading, and that's why she wasn't seeing physical changes in her life yet. The second time she felt it deeply, and her life transformed. Some resist doing the activities the first time, but do them on a later reading, once Grace has opened them up more. You could read it many times, getting more each time.

Others need or want more than the book, so they do the Online Level One or Two Retreat Courses. Others take the Five-Day Silent Retreat for the twelve-hour-a-day immersion in this powerful vortex, the enjoyment, and the daily live Divine Openings.

A Divine Opening may have a delayed effect of days, or even months, depending on what it needs to do within you. For example, you might read the whole book and not feel much at all. Then days, weeks, or months later the Grace has melted through mountains of invisible resistance, and you have a huge awakening, seemingly out of the blue. If you'd wandered back to seeking, you might attribute it to the wrong thing, then it gets really confusing. Seeking and working on yourself reverses the awakening, by definition. You can't be awakened and seeking at the same time. It's like being lost and found, or hot and cold. You can't be both.

Keep using these practices daily until you feel pretty consistently great, and then do maintenance practices in a fun, playful way. Get off that healing-seeking-and-working-on-yourself-treadmill!

The *Thirty Ways To Raise Your Altitude* page near the end of this book serves as a quick guide to staying up and continuing to expand and go higher. There's a Daily Pleasure Practice page, too. Create your own unique practice and refresh it as needed to keep it fun and alive.

Keep playing with it until you've formed new habits and don't need to think about it so much. Then you're free. I don't do much regular practice at all. It's mostly embedded in how I live moment to moment now. Challenges come and go quickly. My mind is sharp and efficient, even post-menopause. My creativity and energy is flowing. I never get stuck for long.

I haven't needed anybody to counsel or work on me spiritually, mentally, or emotionally, nor have I worked on myself, since I developed this work. I'm on the automatic upgrade program, and you can be too. You become more self-correcting, self-healing, and self-guided as you stick to and master this work, but if you need help with a blind spot or area of resistance, we offer options to help you. My body now works better than ever at fifty-seven. I feel fabulous and love hard workouts. I get massages because they feel good and help my body flow this constantly increasing energy. A chiropractor, accupuncturist, and some Divine Openings healers supported me on a couple of physical things.

You may become liberated first, for example, in your relationships, then money, but last in your physical health. The ideal relationship came last for me. It comes when it comes. Complaining that it's not here yet sends you backward, away from it. Appreciate, enjoy, let go! If you're relaxed about when you get there and what it looks like, and are having a great time, you're there now!

Stick With It

IN MY EXPERIENCE with many thousands of people, they rise, stabilize, and maintain their awakening best if they read this book multiple times. I've never seen anyone let it in all at once, no matter how smart or advanced they were. Reading it repeatedly also avoid going back into addictive seeking again before you get fully awake and inner guided.

Your "pipes" expand with each reading, and each time you can let more Grace in. Your conscious mind still requires retraining to allow you to go with the flow of Grace rather than resisting it or contradicting it unknowingly. The mind can tenaciously resist the new way.

The initiation to enlightenment is just a beginning. When you wake up in the morning, you still have sleep in your eyes and you still may not see clearly. So it is with enlightenment. You get the bliss of enlightenment; then you learn to bring it down to earth, to all your relationships, your work, and your life. A process of refinement of your human self occurs.

Enlightenment can happen in a flash, but the awakening into full liberation and retraining of your mind can take time. Our online and live retreats help. They give support to the fragile new sprout of your budding consciousness, while much of the world would trample it. Once you're stabilized, you will be like a mighty oak, a solid support for others. But until then, tend that tender new green shoot with care, giving yourself support and inspiration, nourishment and upliftment.

Before I say this next part, let me be clear: Do whatever you choose. I'm not telling you *what you can and can't do*. Everyone resists that, and they should. I am all about leading you to freedom! If I thought "modality soup" would free you, I'd be recommending every book and seminar out there—and making a fortune doing it. I get weekly offers to use my influence to promote stuff at a profit but I have zero interest in checking all that stuff out, so I can't in good conscience recommend it. Most stuff out there is contradictory to Divine Openings, and trying to do contradictory things together is a recipe for a mess. If, for example, the other stuff has you working on yourself, "healing" your emotions, telling your story, getting "energy work," or someone is "working on you"—you simply won't get the full effect of Divine Openings.

Here's the cowgirl guru again: So many therapies, modalities, and New Age practices don't work—at all. Some work partially, slowly, or temporarily. The definition of insanity is doing the same thing over and over and expecting different results. I've watched a couple of people have some astounding experiences with Divine Openings, get really high and free, then wander off into seeking outside and get lost again. Some can't seem to allow themselves that much power and freedom. Someone said to me after wandering off and then coming back to Divine Openings, "Well, I thought if Divine Openings is this good, more stuff would be even better. It wasn't." If you rely on others to fix, clear, make you feel better or heal your emotions, or to connect you to The Presence, you're not using your Instrument Panel and you remain dependent and outer focused, neglecting the vast resources within you.

I got off that hamster wheel, and I invite you to as well. You have Free Will and you make the decision to wake up fully and be there instead of striving endlessly to get there. Stay with Divine Openings until you are tapped in, clear, inner guided, happy, successful, and questions cease. Then reading a good spiritual poetry book might be inspiring or entertaining, but seeking gets boring.

A Divine Openings session can illuminate a blind spot without giving an ounce of your power away because we'll always point you back to your Large Self. You can let in care and contribution from people in your life, even as you give it to them. An occasional reading with a *high vibration* psychic can help, but watch what you take in, and remember, you created it, so you can take what they say and change it. Most of all, relax, get a life, and enjoy it *now*. Life is for living, not seeking so that someday you can begin to live. Live now.

Faster Isn't Always Better

ALL DIVINE OPENINGS except Mother Divine hugs have an "evolution accelerating" effect, so accelerate only as fast as you can release resistance. In other words, when you resist feeling, letting go, change, and movement in your life, that's like having your foot on the brake, so first, release resistance with Divine Mother hugs, prostrating, or some means before you try to accelerate. Move steadily, but ease up on the need for speed. Having high energy plus high resistance is like stomping on the accelerator and the brake at the same time. It burns up your brakes and your transmission.

In practical terms, this means if you're too wired up, but not moving forward productively, you need to release resistance, not amp up more energy. If life gets chaotic, slow down, and get grounded with mundane physical things like gardening, walking, cleaning, and organizing.

On your second reading of the book, you might skip the formal Divine Openings until you relax, let go, and catch up with the acceleration you already have going. Have more fun, and make sure Divine Openings hasn't become work.

If you're still re-reading this book in a year or two, but you're getting happier and happier, you're on track. When you love your life, it doesn't matter how fast it goes—you are free. Racing toward something all the time is pointless unless your life is joyful.

You cannot feel as deeply when you're running fast, whether it's running toward goals or running away from something. The slower you go, the more you feel. One week, for various reasons I had to slow down and do absolutely nothing for an entire week. It was a revelation. I went even deeper into The Presence, and I thought I was already tapped in, but I felt more, much more. Want to get higher and feel more free? Stop running so fast and slow down so you can be more present. You think you can't afford it, but you can't afford not to.

We created some support pages on the website especially for you readers:

www.DivineOpenings.com/divine-mother-hug - To soothe, steady, and calm you.

www.DivineOpenings.com/spiritual-enlightenment-processes - Helps you apply the book.

www.DivineOpenings.com/spiritual-awakening-articles - Covers many topics not in the book.

Eventually, you'll stop receiving formal Divine Openings except when you feel called occasionally to get one. You'll live and *be* your Large Self, which is the intended result of Divine Openings. Once you can tap in very powerfully on your own, the formal process of receiving a Divine Opening is not necessary. At some point everything falls away and there is just the awakened you, with nothing more to "do" except let the expansion continue, enjoy, and live.

As much as I'm committed to everyone becoming inner guided, over the years I've observed that some people want a teacher and some structure for the long run, and that too is a valid choice. Teachers are specialists in bringing in new energies and guiding people higher. I don't want make having a teacher a bad thing and chase people away, only to have them wander back into fruitless seeking. Do what feels right for you.

Epilogue

IN ITS EARLY years, I updated *Things Are Going Great In My Absence* many times, because Divine Openings constantly expands and evolves. I kept it available only through my website for about three years, then my self-publisher at the time put it on Amazon.com because it was one of their top two selling books. People in over 135 countries were led to it, and only then did I release *Things Are Going Great In My Absence* widely to bookstores. There was never any sense of rush.

My very being is designed and driven (in a good way) to make new Energy/Light/Intelligence accessible to this planet, so rather than updating this book again, as of this edition the unstoppable flow of new material will be added to the online retreats, new books, and audios. At www.DivineOpenings.com/spiritual-awakening-articles, there are forty five free articles, with more added regularly. I particularly recommend *Nineteen Spiritual Myths That Hold You Back.*

www.DivineOpenings.com is a virtual world. It even has its own gravitational pull, evidenced by the number of people who've told me they first found the site when it just popped up on their screen one day—when they weren't touching the computer or searching. Many people make it their home page and start their day reading the daily quote, exploring and soaking up the high resonance that's now their "home frequency." It's a place where you're understood and feel at home.

When *Things Are Going Great In My Absence* was first written, people said they'd never seen anything like it—it was unique and revolutionary. Famous authors, healers, and teachers have adopted some of it in their own work—you'll see pieces of it out there. Yet Divine Openings is most powerful in its pure, *complete,* unadulterated form. The concepts are only ten percent of it—this powerful Grace is ninety percent. In this book and at www.DivineOpenings.com it's presented in it's purest form. Please share it with everyone you love and care about. People are getting free faster and easier than ever.

We love it when you continue to visit the website just to enjoy and add to the vibration, uplift others, be inspired, and participate as community members—we've all made many deep friendships.

Newest developments? When I began singing lessons three years ago I "couldn't carry a tune in a bucket" as my mother would say in her Tennessee way. Well, that changed. Now, there are fifteen of my original songs available on the website, including my favorite, *Here In My Heart.* The theme song for Russell's film *Beautiful Faces* flowed into me—it graces the film's end credits *and* opens my song collection with Tom Hopkins, *Watch Where You Point That Thing,* a joyful, heartfelt, inspiring, rockin' musical ride.

We've raised the possibility of a film about Divine Openings. *Confessions Of A Cowgirl Guru* will be a laugh-out-loud humor DVD as well as a book. Another dream is to sing live, and the offers are there—I'm just surfing the joy of it right now while busy with other things. I'll keep merrily expanding and evolving (but not working on myself ever again) till the day Russell and I consciously, ecstatically choose to depart the planet.

Always Love,
Lola

Thirty Ways To Raise Your Altitude

Notice that these all feel good and *none of them are work!* Do them for joy, and not just to solve problems. They help you retrain yourself to operate at a higher frequency. There is no limit to how high you can go and how good you can feel. Use them in your Daily Practice.

Be patient, consistent, and easy about this if you have practiced resistance for a long time. Some of these methods will work starting from anywhere on the Altimeter. Others will work best when you are already flying fairly high. Try different ones until one works.

1. **Breathe for pleasure:** Sit or lie down. Smile, and arch your back slightly as you inhale for five counts, and bend your spine gently forward as you breathe out for five counts. Silently say "yessss"on the inhale and breathe "ahhh" on the exhale. Breathe easily for five to fifteen minutes.

2. **Soothe yourself:** Move energy up step by step on a subject by telling yourself a better story about that subject. Be soft on yourself. "Where I am is where I am. I can get anywhere from wherever I am. This is temporary. Everything changes. Things always work out."

3. **Have a Date With The Divine:** Silence. No people, television, telephone, computer or email.

4. **Fork in the road:** Choose the better-feeling thought or action and feel the immediate relief.

5. **Turn your body:** Get up and turn your whole body in a different direction. Turn away from what you don't want, toward what you *do* want, and feel the difference in your body.

6. **Choose your focus:** In every moment, choose only past, present, or future thoughts that feel good when you think about them.

7. **Move your body:** Exercise and act out each emotion to raise you from where you are to several steps up. Several steps up are plenty. Stabilize. *Download some of Lola's Divine Music at www.DivineOpenings.com/about-music*

8. **Daydream:** For entertainment only! This is not work. What you want is already "given," created, and done. Your job is to vibrate, think, and feel in harmony with it so it can materialize.

9. **Add humor:** Make the day or the daydream humorous—it's your show!

10. **Rave about it!** Think of everything there is to appreciate about a person or subject, yourself or your life in general, and rave on and on about it. Do this silently or out loud.

11. **Dive in:** Drop the story about it. Say "yes" to the unwanted feeling as you breathe into it. Any feeling fully felt rises.

12. **Prostrate:** Lay it down at the feet of The Divine. Breathe for pleasure until you feel a lift.

13. **Dream Intention:** Make a list of everything you want, put it to dream assignment and let go. Sleep easy, knowing it's being handled. Follow what feels good the next day and watch for subtle guidance in any form. Drop any timetable and don't take score. It's done.

14. **Put it on the God List:** Make a long list of everything you need and give the whole list over to The Presence. The Presence already knows. This just has you let go and get out of the way!

15. **Take a break:** Take your focus completely off the difficult subject and do something that feels good instead.

16. **Vacation:** Take a vacation or a mini-vacation and let go of "work." No phones, no computers, no effort. Break your routine entirely and just let go and relax.

17. **Pet pampering:** Play with your pets. Feel how joyful they are.

18. **Laugh:** Look for something funny and light—jokes, funny book, friend or movie.

19. **Ask your Large Self:** "What do you know and feel about this?" "What would work better?" "How could I experience this differently?" "What amazing development is next for me?"

20. **Ask your Large Self:** "How could I choose being happy instead of being right?"

21. **Ask your Large Self:** "What is my next little step?" Take that step without question.

22. **Take score of wins.** Focus on how far you've come and what has worked out.

23. **Don't take score:** Delay taking score of yet-un-materialized things, or things that didn't work. Say, "Next!" or "It's still coming! My job is to raise my altitude and feel good about it."

24. **Feel good first:** Do two things that feel good to you, then do your "must do's" afterward. Luxuriate in the bed before you rise. Take a bath, walk, sing, garden, etc.

25. **Have it now:** Put yourself in the feeling of "having it now." Gather information, visit places physically and "test drive" any desire you have that feels too far away.

26. **Claim your power:** At each little elevation say, "I created just a little relief! If I can do that I can do anything! All it takes is one step like that at a time."
—When unwanted manifestations show up, say, "I created that! How powerful I am!"
—When things you do want show up, say, "I created that! How powerful I am!"

27. **Be happy now:** You think being somewhere else or having things be different will make you happy. Take the short cut and be happy now. Then Law of Attraction can give you more of it.

28. **Give up control:** Mind your own business. Let other people, the world, and things outside you be, do, and have whatever they choose. Choose your reality independent of that, knowing that no one can create in your reality or hold you back—only you can.

29. **Easy button:** Hit your "easy button" every time something goes well or comes easy! Order them online at Staples.com. Give them to friends!

30. **Breathe-For-Pleasure Meditation:** There is no resistance while you're not thinking. Sit. Smile slightly. Minutely arch your back as you inhale, and bend your spine forward a tiny bit as you exhale. In your mind, say "yes" on the inhale, and "ahhh" on the exhale. Let all thoughts go on by. If you lose focus on the breath, gently refocus. Make it a special date with your Beloved Presence in The Silence. Breathe for pleasure for five to fifteen minutes.

Sample Daily Pleasure Practice

Morning:
1. **Breathe-For-Pleasure Meditation:** There is no resistance while you're not thinking. Sit. Smile slightly. Minutely arch your back a bit as you inhale, and bend your spine forward a tiny bit as you exhale. In your mind, say "yes" on the inhale, and "ahhh," on the exhale. Enjoy for five to fifteen minutes.

2. **Rave about it:** Focus on appreciating yourself, everything, and everyone you can for five minutes.

3. **Daydream:** Playfully imagine how you want your day to go or how you want it to feel, just for entertainment. (Don't take score if it doesn't immediately go that way. Take score only on what did go well.) Pleasantly anticipate how you'd like each individual activity to go before you begin. Line up the energy, and action flows smoother.

4. **Feel good:** Do things that feel good—listen or move to Lola's Divine Music (found at www.DivineOpenings.com) or others, sing, garden, take a bath, take a walk, pet your cat. You'll be more productive. You can always feel even better.

As You Go About Your Day:
1. **Inspired action:** Do the actions you are inspired to do first. Act when it feels guided, when your altitude is high on that subject, unless there is an absolute deadline like taxes.

2. **Take breaks:** Sit quietly and breathe for pleasure. Especially when it seems you must rush or work harder: Stop. Tune inward and get in alignment with your Large Self. Feel your guidance system's input.

Evening:
1. **Feel good:** Do something that feels good to you.

2. **Move your body and play:** Dance, walk, sing, run with the dog, bike, or swim. Wiggle, jump, laugh, be goofy. Moving the body in unusual ways unsticks the mind.

3. **Savor:** Luxuriate in smells, sights, sensations, touch, and sounds. Enjoy sensual moments wherever you find or create them.

Before bed:
1. **Rave:** Focus on appreciating yourself, everything, and everyone you can for five minutes.

2. **Breathe-For-Pleasure Meditation:** Sit. Smile slightly. Minutely arch your back a bit as you inhale, and bow your spine forward a tiny bit as you breathe out. Breathe effortlessly for five minutes.

3. **Set Dream Intentions.** Relax, smile slightly, snuggle in, and let go.

Add your own favorites. Update it often.

ADDITIONAL SERVICES AND RESOURCES:
Go to www.DivineOpenings.com and subscribe to our newsletter. You'll receive inspirational articles, gifts, updates, and invitations to events. To stop receiving emails, just click "unsubscribe." We never, ever send email to people who didn't subscribe and double confirm. Thank you.

Special free support pages for readers of this book:
www.DivineOpenings.com/spiritual-awakening-articles
www.DivineOpenings.com/divine-mother-hug
www.DivineOpenings.com/spiritual-enlightenment-processes

Check the website often for new audios, videos, courses, articles, features, and events.

Download Lola's Original Music at www.DivineOpenings.com. The Presence moves through Lola to create inspired music in all genres, dance, pop, blues, to spiritual.

Divine Openings Online Retreat Courses: Level 1, Level 2, and Jumping The Matrix, First Aid For Special Topics, Advanced Healing, The Art of Sex and Love. www.DivineOpenings.com.

Live Retreats: Get on the newsletter list to hear about Five Day Retreats in U.S. and abroad.

Divine Openings accepts donations and tithes. See Donate button in site menu.

Lola's Art: Visit www.DivineOpenings.com. Order Divine Art, from 8x10 high-resolution prints to poster-size reproductions of paintings. Greeting cards with Divine Energy are great gifts. Commissioned Paintings: With Divine Energy channeled just for you.
Prints on Paper or Canvas: Most artworks on the website are available by special order.

Russell Martin, Lola's love, makes beautiful films that matter, and writes books. Visit *Say Yes Quickly Productions* (named after a line in a Rumi poem) at www.syqproductions.net.

OTHER BOOKS FROM LOLA JONES:

Dating To Change Your Life makes dating fun, transforming your life in the process. Get happy and find your partner faster. This book is pre-Divine Openings, but it's good—and it's funny.

Divine Openings Quotes is a beautiful book of wisdom; heart-opening, funny, surprising.

BOOKS COMING SOON:

Watch Where You Point That Thing: Mastering Your Power Of Intention—Corresponds with Divine Openings Level Two Online.

Confessions Of A Cowgirl Guru—A humor collection inspired by Lola's life, loves, and observations about the holistic culture and the metaphysical life. Get on the newsletter list and watch the website.

More comments from readers. There are thousands more on the website:

Awareness of how I've been resistant to receiving came up strongly. I asked God to soften me and then that 'download' happened again immediately, and He held me and showed me exactly what to do. I've never experienced automatic writing before—what an awesome experience. Thank you for helping me remember my way home as I'd gotten lost lately. —Blessings to you, Michelle Wolff

So much has happened so fast that I can barely even articulate it. I am just so grateful that I found your work on the net. Why, why, why doesn't Oprah know about you? Your work is the obvious next step to the Tolle stuff because of its practical, down to earth, how-to accessibility. I can just imagine a Divine Opening on the Oprah show! I'm sending you love. —Donna Wetterstrand, Canada

I just listened to your trauma and abuse audio on the Diving In series, and it is one of the most exquisite pieces of therapy I've ever heard. I've been in this field for these many years and nothing I have seen, heard, done, or delivered myself even comes close. Another WOW! —Donna

The energy was incredible. I had to go slower than one opening a week—I found myself moving very quickly. I would look back at things I did just a week or two ago and say to myself, why did I handle it that way when I know it could have been handled like this…. then I realized that a week or two ago I wasn't in the place I am now! I feel less stressed, more like I am floating through life— not all the time, but more and more. Thank you! —Eleanor

As you gave the Divine Opening (on the phone) I was aware of my feet . . . and I saw in my mind's eye, the hands of Jesus washing them. The sensation of a breeze softly blowing around my ankles and feet started and continues even now, seven hours later. Sweet! —Julie, Arizona

I've had some significant movement. I love your unshakable faith, your playfulness, that you are a 'powerhouse renegade,' and how your wisdom cuts through to profound truth. —Much Love, Naraya

Lola, everything I want . . . It's not coming . . . It's already HERE! I just have to KEEP letting it in! IT feels so amazing. —Love, Nicole

Many times I felt like people who I love were inside me and I could feel their love for me, also. —Ana

My body is changing from within. Sometimes I can't eat foods I used to like, and I don't want those foods. So I am losing a bit of weight now too. —Edith

Thanks for keeping up with me, as I probably need supervision (just kidding.) Well, after much groundwork and trial and error, everything is falling into place for my business. I'm retired, but like all intense people, retirement means just having enough free time to start another business. I've searched for a teacher of my kind of spirituality. I know this is "it." Nothing else has ever felt this way for me. —All my love and gratitude, Kathy

I gave the book to my mom in Georgia who is 78. She called me yesterday all excited about her first Divine Opening. What she explained to me was that she felt a pulse run through her whole body, even in her fingertips. Then she saw a light around a black hole, she explained that things were going into the black hole really fast, and then it closed up and disappeared. It is going to be fun to keep sharing these experiences with my Mom. I am giving a book to my daughter Rachel, 24. You will be touching the lives of 3 generations in my family. —Carey Waters

My husband and I have a code word—"the Book"—we say it when one of us is crabby or aggravated. Then we smile and laugh a little because we both know what it means. Sincerely and with love, —Julie

CPSIA information can be obtained at www.ICGtesting.com
Printed in the USA
LVOW090227191112

307915LV00006B/3/P

EBCFAPR